Religion and Ethics in the Neonatal Intensive Care Unit

Religion and Ethics in the Neonatal Intensive Care Unit

Edited by

RONALD M. GREEN AND GEORGE A. LITTLE

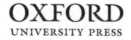

OXFORD
UNIVERSITY PRESS

Oxford University Press is a department of the University of Oxford. It furthers
the University's objective of excellence in research, scholarship, and education
by publishing worldwide. Oxford is a registered trade mark of Oxford University
Press in the UK and certain other countries.

Published in the United States of America by Oxford University Press
198 Madison Avenue, New York, NY 10016, United States of America.

© Oxford University Press 2019

Library of Congress Cataloging-in-Publication Data
Names: Green, Ronald Michael, editor. | Little, George A. (George Alexiy),
1939– editor.
Title: Religion and ethics in the neonatal intensive care unit /
[edited by] Ronald M. Green and George A. Little.
Description: New York, NY : Oxford University Press, [2019] |
Includes bibliographical references.
Identifiers: LCCN 2019012595 | ISBN 9780190636852 (hardback) |
ISBN 9780190636869 (Updf) | ISBN 9780190636876 (Epub) |
ISBN 9780190636883 (online)
Subjects: | MESH: Intensive Care, Neonatal—ethics | Intensive Care Units, Neonatal—ethics |
Family-centered care | Religion and Medicine | Clinical Decision-Making—ethics
Classification: LCC RJ253.5 | NLM WS 421 | DDC 174.2/989201—dc23
LC record available at https://lccn.loc.gov/2019012595

1 3 5 7 9 8 6 4 2

Printed by Sheridan Books, Inc., United States of America

Contents

Acknowledgments

This book is the result of more than five years of work in cooperation with the annual Gravens Conference on the Environment of Care for High Risk Newborns, where each of our chapters began as a session presentation. From the start, the leadership of the conference committed to supporting a multi-year examination of the teachings of the major world religious traditions on the status and care of premature or sick full-term newborns. Year by year, attendees at the conference and our sessions enhanced our understanding of the issues with their insightful comments and observations, including suggestions for future presenters in our series. We extend a special word of thanks to Bobbi Rose for her management of the logistics and funding.

Thanks, too, to Dartmouth College and Dartmouth-Hitchcock Medical Center for the support over many years that helped foster our collaboration.

Lucy Randall and Peter Ohlin at Oxford University Press were supportive of this effort from our first mention of it to them early in our work.

Finally, we would like to express special thanks to Kier Olsen DeVries, who edited each chapter and served as the organizing center for all our efforts. This project could not have been successfully completed without Kier's support.

Contributors

Zahra Ayubi, Ph.D., is an assistant professor of religion at Dartmouth College. She specializes in gender in classical and contemporary Islamic ethics. Her scholarship is a feminist engagement with the Islamic intellectual tradition that seeks to advance understandings of the ways that gender is constructed in Islamic philosophy and operates in historical and contemporary transnational Muslim communities.

Swasti Bhattacharyya, Ph.D., R.N., is professor of philosophy and religion at Buena Vista University. Trained as a registered nurse, she is the author of *Magical Progeny, Modern Technology: A Hindu Bioethics of Assisted Reproductive Technology* and a number of articles on ethics, religion, social justice, and pedagogy. She is Director of BVU's Gender and Women's Studies program. Additionally, she serves on the board of the Peace and Justice Studies Association and is actively involved with the American Academy of Religion.

Ronald Cole-Turner, M.Div., Ph.D., holds the H. Parker Sharp Chair in Theology and Ethics at Pittsburgh Theological Seminary and is a research fellow of the Research Institute for Theology and Religion, University of South Africa. He is a founding member and a vice president of the International Society for Science and Religion. His most recent book is a study of human evolution and its theological significance, entitled *The End of Adam and Eve: Theology and the Science of Human Origins* (2016).

Elliot N. Dorff, Rabbi, Ph.D., is rector and Distinguished Service Professor of Philosophy at American Jewish University and visiting professor at University of California Los Angeles School of Law. He has served on three federal commissions on medical issues (the distribution of health care, reducing sexually transmitted infections, and research on human subjects) and currently serves on the State of California's ethics committee for stem cell research in the state. *Matters of Life and Death: A Jewish Approach to Modern Medical Ethics* is one of the thirteen books he has written on Jewish thought, law, and ethics, and *Jews and Genes: The Genetic Future in Contemporary Jewish Thought* (co-edited with Laurie Zoloth) is among the additional fourteen books he has edited or co-edited.

Erin Dufault-Hunter, Ph.D., is assistant professor of Christian ethics at Fuller Theological Seminary. She teaches, speaks, and publishes about implications that our embodiment has for the moral life, particularly among Christians. Her books include *The Transformative Power of Faith: A Narrative Approach to Conversion* and *Shalom, Health, and Healing: Frontiers and Challenges in Christian Health Care Missions* (co-edited with Bryant Myers and Isaac Voss).

Ronald M. Green, Ph.D., is Professor Emeritus for the Study of Ethics and Human Values at Dartmouth College. He was a member of Dartmouth's Department of Religion from 1969 to 2015 and is a member of the Department of Community and Family Medicine at

Dartmouth's Geisel School of Medicine. He is the author of nine books, editor of four, and author of more than 170 articles in theoretical and applied ethics. His most recent books include *Babies by Design: The Ethics of Genetic Choice* and *Suffering and Bioethics* (co-edited with Nathan Palpant).

George A. Little, M.D., is an active emeritus professor of pediatrics and of obstetrics-gynecology at Dartmouth's Geisel School of Medicine. An academic clinician and sub-specialist in neonatology, he is widely known for domestic and global contributions, including many publications. His special interests include maternal and child health outcomes, systems of perinatal care, family-centered care, and medical decision making. Leadership responsibilities include being a board member since the 1987 inception of the Gravens Conference on the Environment of Care for High Risk Newborns where chapters of this volume have been presented.

M. Therese Lysaught, Ph.D., is a professor at the Neiswanger Institute of Bioethics and Health Policy at Loyola University Chicago's Stritch School of Medicine and at the Institute of Pastoral Studies. She has also served as a visiting scholar with the Catholic Health Association. Her books include *Caritas in Communion: Theological Foundations of Catholic Health Care, On Moral Medicine: Theological Perspectives on Medical Ethics,* 3rd edition (co-edited with Joseph Kotva), *Gathered for the Journey: Moral Theology in Catholic Perspective* (co-edited with David M. McCarthy), and *Catholic Bioethics and Social Justice* (co-edited with Michael McCarthy).

Maureen Trudelle Schwarz, Ph.D., is professor emerita of anthropology in the Maxwell School of Citizenship and Public Affairs at Syracuse University. She was the founding director of the Native American and Indigenous Studies Program at Syracuse University. She is the author of *Blood and Voice: The Life-Courses of Navajo Women Ceremonial Practitioners,* and *Navajo Lifeways: Contemporary Issues, Ancestral Knowledge.*

Patrick T. Smith, Ph.D., is associate research professor of theological ethics and bioethics at Duke University Divinity School. He is also a senior fellow for the Kenan Institute of Ethics, Duke University and associate faculty with the Trent Center for Bioethics, Humanities, and History of Medicine, Duke University School of Medicine. He previously served as the ethics coordinator for Angela Hospice Care Center (Michigan) and core faculty for Harvard's Center for Bioethics. He has specific interests in the relationship of bioethics with social ethics, and the interface of hospice/palliative care with moral philosophy, theology, religion, and spirituality.

Vincent C. Smith, M.D., MPH., is the Division Chief of Neonatology at Boston Medical Center and associate professor of pediatrics at Boston University Medical School. He is a co-chair for the Gravens Conference on the Environment of Care for High Risk Newborns. Dr. Smith is a graduate of Texas A&M University, Stanford University School of Medicine, and the Harvard School of Public Health. Dr. Smith serves as the medical director for the American Academy of Pediatrics' Fetal Alcohol Spectrum Disorders Program. He is a member of the Board of Directors of the National Perinatal Association. He is also an active member of the Massachusetts Medical Society, Society for Pediatric Research, and Maternal Child Health Advisory Committee at the Harvard School of Public Health. In addition to parental NICU discharge readiness, his professional interests also include families affected by substance use.

Karma Lekshe Tsomo, Ph.D., is professor of Buddhist Studies at the University of San Diego, where she teaches Buddhist Thought and Culture, Death and Dying, and World Religions. She holds a doctorate in Comparative Philosophy from the University of Hawai'i at Mānoa, with a dissertation on "Death and Identity in China and Tibet." She is the author of *Into the Jaws of Yama, Lord of Death: Buddhism, Bioethics, and Death.* Her research interests include Buddhist feminist philosophy, Buddhism and bioethics, Buddhist social theory, concepts of death and afterlife, and Buddhist transnationalism.

Juzer M. Tyebkhan, MBBS, FRCPC, is a neonatologist and associate clinical professor in the Department of Pediatrics, Division of Neonatal-Perinatal Care (NICU) at the Stollery Children's Hospital in Edmonton, Alberta, Canada. His areas of special interest include developmental care, NIDCAP (Newborn Individualized Developmental Care and Assessment Program), preterm infant follow-up, and family-centered care.

Gerald R. Winslow, Ph.D., is professor of religion at Loma Linda University, where he also serves as director of the university's Center for Christian Bioethics and is the founding director of the Institute for Health Policy and Leadership. His books include *Triage and Justice* and *Facing Limits: Ethics and Healthcare for the Elderly* (co-edited with James Walters).

Introduction

Ronald M. Green and George A. Little

During the past two decades, two difficult British biomedical cases involving decision making about sick newborns drew the world's attention. The first occurred in 2000 and involved conjoined twins, Jodie and Mary, whose separation for the sake of Jodie's survival entailed the death of the medically more compromised Mary. The second case extended from 2016 into 2017 and had at its center Charles Matthew William Gard. Charlie was born with a rare genetic disease (mitochondrial DNA depletion syndrome, or MDDS) that causes progressive brain damage and muscle failure and that usually leads to death in infancy. Drawing on the hope offered by an unproven medical treatment, Charlie's parents engaged in—and finally lost—a protracted legal battle with Charlie's medical caregivers, who had concluded that further treatment for Charlie was futile and only likely to prolong the infant's suffering.

Each of these cases pitted parents' wishes against the professional judgments of medical professionals. Each involved complex ethical issues that finally had to be adjudicated in the courts.[1] Each also took place against a background of powerful religious beliefs motivating the parents or their supporters. This was evident in the case of the conjoined twins, whose parents, drawing on their understanding of their Catholic faith, regarded the surgical separation of the weaker twin in order to save her sister's life as tantamount to deliberate and wrongful killing. In the case of Charlie Gard, his parents' conviction that Charlie's life must be saved at all costs was reinforced when religious leaders, including Pope Francis, entered the fray on their side. Amid the controversy, they documented their celebration of their son's baptism and showed him clutching a pendant of St. Jude, the Catholic figure most often associated with hospitals and medical care.[2]

These two are extreme cases. Parents' religious convictions only rarely lead them into overt conflict with their medical caregivers. But religious beliefs often profoundly influence parents' interaction with healthcare professionals in the neonatal intensive care unit (NICU) or pediatric intensive care setting when difficult ethical decisions have to be made about an infant's care. The role of religion in shaping parents' thinking becomes particularly relevant in those NICUs committed to family-centered care. Such care requires a partnership between parents and caregivers and, whenever possible, shared decision making. In cases of infants with conditions marked by high mortality, morbidity, or "great suffering," family-centered care affirms the right of parents "to make decisions regarding aggressive treatment for their infant."[3]

There is evidence that religious beliefs strongly influence families' treatment decisions about their loved ones, especially when difficult life-and-death moral choices must be made. For example, one study of the families of adult cancer patients found that family members expressing strong religious convictions were twice as likely as more secular individuals to want "all measures" to extend their loved one's life.[4] Another study looked explicitly at the NICU setting. It reported the answers of parents of term and preterm infants to the question of whether they would prefer to see their child die rather than face "severe global disability." The Hong Kong setting of the study, with a large proportion of the local population being atheists, provided the rare opportunity to examine the effects of religion—in particular, Christianity and frequency of worship—on parents' attitudes. The study found that religious parents who worshipped regularly were on average five times more likely to prefer severe global disability to death for their infant. It concluded, "Regular parental religious worship was positively associated with a significantly increased probability of deciding to save the infant at all costs."[5] Still another study documented the difficulties experienced by neonatal nurses when caring for an extremely premature baby whose parents unrealistically hold on to hope and their belief in divine intervention and a miracle.[6]

Although the Hong Kong study focused mostly on religious parents who were self-identified as Christian, not all Christians advocate preserving life at all costs. Moreover, other religious traditions, such as Judaism, Islam, Hinduism, or Buddhism, can have very different views about newborn care. The understanding that parents' religious beliefs and identification significantly influence their decision making about their sick newborn thus raises an important question: What are the teachings of the world's major religious traditions about the status and care of the newborn?

Surprisingly, this question has rarely been addressed in the literature of bioethics. Although there are many discussions of religious teachings about the fetus and abortion or about end-of-life care for adults or older pediatric patients, there are few discussions of religious teachings about the care of premature or sick newborns.[7] Yet such teachings, whether invoked by families on the basis of their culturally inherited understandings or offered by trained pastoral counselors, clearly play a role in shaping many parents' response to difficult treatment decisions for a sick newborn.

In 2013, after being approached by the editors of this volume, the leadership of the annual Gravens Conference on the Environment of Care for High Risk Newborns committed to supporting a multi-year examination of the teachings of the major world religious traditions on the status and care of premature or sick full-term newborns. The immediate goal was to inform Gravens attendees, who comprise a range of NICU professionals—physicians, nurses, social workers, pastoral counselors, architects, and administrators—as well as parents of NICU graduates. A long-term objective was to gather these presentations in the form of chapters for an edited volume that could serve as a resource for neonatal professionals as well as a support for parents of NICU patients working with their caregivers and seeking, perhaps with their religious counselors, a better understanding of their own tradition's teachings. The conference presentations and book project fit well with the larger goal of the Gravens Conference of fostering improved care and outcomes for newborns.[8]

Accordingly, in the four years from 2014 to 2017, a special two-hour session of each annual Gravens Conference was dedicated to presentations by leading bioethicists and scholars of the world's major religious traditions. Several of these presenters had firsthand knowledge of the NICU environment, whether as a parent, medical professional, or clinical consultant. The chapters in this book are the result of this work. Together, they offer new and unparalleled insights into the teachings of major world religious traditions about the newborn. Traditions covered include Judaism; Roman Catholicism; evangelical, denominational (mainstream), and African American Protestantism; Islam; Hinduism; Buddhism; Seventh-day Adventism; and Navajo religions. Most of these traditions have a global presence, and all are represented among parents and staff in North American NICU settings. The topics treated for each tradition are comprehensive. They comprise each tradition's understanding of the moral status and moral claims of the newborn, including infants born at the threshold of viability; the ethical obligations of parents and caregivers to infants facing a high risk of mortality and morbidity or severe lifelong disability; when, if ever, it is ethically permissible to withhold or withdraw treatment from a medically imperiled newborn or one facing death in infancy; religious understandings of parental authority for decision making, including the respective roles of mothers and fathers; and the tradition's ritual requirements surrounding childbirth and the handling of an infant's body during treatment or after death.

Although contributors were asked in their presentation and writings to address this range of questions, each chapter is an original reflection, interpreting the challenges involved in newborn care within the framework of each tradition's deepest religious beliefs, ethical values, and ritual practices. While offering normative moral guidance for caregivers, pastoral counselors, or parents, therefore, these chapters are also original philosophical and spiritual reflections on each tradition's understanding of the ethical and spiritual meaning of life's fragile beginnings.

Rather than reiterating the contents of each chapter, it may be helpful here to indicate some of these chapters' overarching lessons. What broad insights might readers develop from this study? What are the important "take-home" points that NICU caregivers in particular might gather from reading this book? We identify at least six major insights that these chapters provide.

A first insight, supported by chapter after chapter, is that each religious tradition is far from monolithic. This is true first because each tradition contains a variety of normative moral views and offers different permissible approaches to hard choices. As the chapters on Judaism by Rabbi Elliot Dorff, on Islam by Zahra Ayubi and Juzer Tyebkhan, and on Hinduism by Swasti Bhattacharyya reveal, multiple strands of authority or sub-traditions mark each of these traditions. When dealing with a Jewish family, for example, much depends on whether they identify as Orthodox or Reform. In the case of Islam, a family's beliefs will be influenced by the teachings of the branch of the tree of Islam to which the family belongs. Thus, the Muslim communities treated by Ayubi and Tyebkhan share many issues of concern to Muslims generally, including a desire for alternatives to alcohol- and porcine-derived treatments or medications, a reluctance to use banked breast milk because of kinship issues, a resistance to autopsy, and a desire for prompt burial. But somewhat differently from many other Muslim communities, the Shi'a Dawoodi Bohra Muslim sub-community that Tyebkhan discusses has a living spiritual leader, the Da'i, who serves as the decider of moral questions or treatment choices. Appreciating subtle differences like this can play an important role in working with a Muslim family.

Even a religious tradition with a single moral teaching authority, such as Roman Catholicism, exhibits a plurality of interpretations on matters such as withdrawing or withholding treatment. Although Catholic leaders spoke out with one voice in the cases of the conjoined twins and Charlie Gard, Catholicism's strong emphasis on the role of individual conscience permitted many Catholics to disagree. Knowing what the Magisterium, or Catholic teachings authority, has to say can be useful in dealing with a devout Catholic family, but it may not be the final word on their thinking.

This diversity within traditions is further amplified by the sheer complexity of modern societies, the growing emphasis on personal autonomy, and the omnipresence of secular attitudes. As Therese Lysaught, speaking from within the Catholic tradition, observes, "simply because a patient or family identifies with a particular religious tradition, that does not mean that the teachings, beliefs, and practices of that tradition necessarily influence their actions and decisions or influence the actions and decisions of all members of a tradition in the same way."[9] Similarly, Zahra Ayubi, in her treatment of Muslim families, reminds us that "Muslims are not their scripture. That is, they may or may not follow scripture or law."[10] The take-home here is that while it is helpful to have familiarity with the teachings of a family's professed religion, caregivers must never assume that parents or families adhere strictly to those teachings or are necessarily guided by the advice of pastoral counselors. Drawing on his experience as a neonatologist, Vincent Smith makes this point in his Afterword to this book when he reminds us that "while it helps to understand what the family's belief system is, it is important to keep an open mind and not assume that one knows the family's wishes and preferences based solely on knowledge of their belief system."[11] The appropriate stance of healthcare professionals assisting families, therefore, is what Bhattacharyya calls "cultural humility," the willingness to "prepare ourselves to listen so we can hear the hopes, fears, and needs of our patients and their families."[12]

A second insight furnished by these chapters is that the teachings of all these traditions are very much works in progress. As Rabbi Dorff points out, the classical teachers of Judaism could never have imagined the possibilities of resuscitation and treatment afforded by modern NICU care. This has forced modern religious scholars in every tradition to seek guidance by analogy from ancient stories, examples, or laws. In some cases, received teachings have left a tradition unable to accommodate to technical innovation, as Maureen Trudelle Schwarz observes in connection with the wary attitudes of the Navajo community about cardiopulmonary resuscitation.[13] It can be expected, therefore, that traditions will evolve as they encounter new and challenging developments in newborn care. Roman Catholicism illustrates this in its current wrestling with the limits to the ethical requirement of providing artificial nutrition and hydration.[14] Once again, cultural humility is in order, as is a willingness of healthcare professionals to keep parents and religious teachers informed of the meaning, possibilities, and limits of medical developments. The prophylactic administration of immunoglobulin to Rh-negative women as a means of reducing the need for blood transfusions in cases of Rh sensitization in children born to Jehovah's Witness parents[15] reveals both the rapidity of change and the importance of collaborative efforts to solve problems posed by religious and value conflict.

A leading ethical issue of NICU care today is whether it is appropriate to pursue aggressive treatment for a newborn experiencing extreme prematurity or severe illness with accompanying morbidity. A third insight offered by these chapters is that in answering this question, all these traditions take a middle ground. Several of these traditions differ on precisely at what point before birth human life in a moral sense begins. Some differ, too, on the question of when following birth the infant is ritually entered into the community. But despite these differences, all regard the newborn, however premature, as a human patient deserving of strenuous medical efforts. This is especially true when the child can survive to a state of reasonable health, even if with some disability. At the same time, almost all these traditions permit either the withholding or withdrawal of treatment when that treatment only forestalls death and causes extreme suffering and disability. In other words, none of these traditions is "vitalist," holding that mere biological life must be sustained at all costs. It is certainly not the case that the withdrawal of life support would never be permitted, or that all possible lifesaving treatments must be attempted regardless of complications. But at the same time, all these traditions also appear to oppose the opposite extreme to vitalism: active euthanasia, "mercy killing" in the form of the intentional taking of the life of a suffering or dying person.

These traditions arrive at this middle ground in various ways. In some cases, such as the Catholic teaching of proportionate means, the tradition is based on a well-developed body of moral reflection. In others, more spiritually based resources play a role, such as the Islamic teaching that God alone determines the infant's fate, the Navajo teaching that each person has a predetermined life span that cannot be changed, or the Hindu and Buddhist belief in reincarnation, which, as Swasti Bhattacharyya and Karma Lekshe Tsomo observe, leads many adherents to view death in infancy as a brief and transitory moment followed by rebirth. Families in the Dawoodi Bohra Muslim community will be instructed by the views of their spiritual leader, but as Juzer Tyebkhan observes, "It is certainly not the case that the withdrawal of life support treatment would never be permitted, or that all possible lifesaving treatments must be attempted regardless of complications."[16] Patrick Smith, speaking out of the black Christian tradition, observes that "death is not final" but is followed by "the great hope" of resurrection, adding that "to embrace this earthly life as the highest good or as something that has absolute value to be hung onto at all costs can easily slide into a form of idolatry."[17] At the same time, Smith warns that the use of quality of life arguments to support active euthanasia runs counter to this tradition's strong affirmation of the equal value of all lives. A treatment may not be worthwhile, says Smith, but whatever their quality, individual lives always are.

Caregivers can expect that parents belonging to all the traditions examined here will be open to ceasing or withdrawal of care in desperate cases and will favor palliative efforts such as comfort care and pain relief for the dying infant, but also that they will be correspondingly opposed to anything perceived as deliberately causing or hastening a child's death.

A fourth take-home suggested by these chapters is the repeated affirmation of the importance of religious ritual and the presence of community associated with it. Erin Dufault-Hunter offers one of the most poignant examples of this when she describes the dedication, naming, and anointing ritual prepared by her Mennonite community for the parents of a dying Trisomy-13 infant. This ritual, says Dufault-Hunter, expressed both the parents' and the community's love for a child whose limited future was fully acknowledged. Similar ritual events, often involving members of the larger family or religious community, are mentioned in chapter after chapter, from rituals as simple as a mother's formalized handshake greeting to her newborn among the Navajo to a full baptism ritual among mainline Protestants. As Ronald Cole-Turner emphasizes, mainstream

Protestants long ago rejected the idea that baptism is required for a child's eternal salvation, but the ritual, even when performed for a dying infant, is an assertion of the value of that child's life: "It is an act of faith in the gift-like reality of the birth despite the obvious and painful truth of the reality that this gift is not at all the gift that was expected."[18]

Therese Lysaught reminds us that a deep emotional commitment to ritual or sacramental practices may persist even among individuals or families who have abandoned active religious involvement or identity. As she observes, "Sacramental practices, augmented by artifacts of material culture (such as images of Our Lady of Guadalupe for Latino/a Catholics or the Sacred Heart of Jesus for Catholics of European descent), are critical resources for many Catholics in times of illness, discernment, and death. When faced with a medical crisis, even Catholics who seldom attend Mass—or who may not have set foot in a church for decades—will instinctively turn to the sacraments and rites of the Church for comfort, for strength, for tradition, or for reasons unknown even to them."[19]

In this vein, Patrick Smith points to the ritual importance of active prayer, song, and reading of the Bible, which are likely to be practiced by African American Christians in the NICU. Although prayer for the healing of an infant with Trisomy 18, Tay-Sachs disease, or Lesch-Nyhan syndrome may alarm NICU staff, such prayer should not be understood as an obstacle to the family's participation in making important decisions about their severely impaired infant. In many cases, Smith observes, prayer for healing plays a ritualized role. It is "an affirmation of faith that these issues are in the hands of God."[20]

The ethical take-home here for NICU caregivers is that efforts should always be made to accommodate the ritual and communal needs of religious parents. This can include parents, accompanied by staff, taking a baby outside the building to open space for withdrawal of care or comfort care and dying. Sometimes accommodations may prove difficult or impossible, as in the case of the Hindu devotional or blessing ritual (puja), which involves the use of an open flame. But even when accommodating parents' ritual needs is demanding, it should be regarded as an important part of the care and caring offered by NICU staff. As Dufault-Hunter observes in connection with the dedication ritual she describes, "One cannot underestimate the value of the staff's willingness to secure time and space for this gathering. It indicates how crucial cooperation and adaptability in hospital settings can be for people of faith, especially when such rituals require a community to witness to it."[21]

While on the topic of staff, we should mention that NICU caregivers often have faith-based values of their own. Staff members bring religious and moral values to their work, and the relation of these values to parents' religious needs should not be overlooked. Staff may sometimes wish to participate in (or absent themselves from) activities related to parents' religious needs. Caregivers' involvement in prayer is a complex issue that arises in this context and one that must be resolved by each professional on a personal basis.[22]

A fifth insight offered by these chapters is that NICU caregivers should seek to develop awareness of the contexts to which their patients' families belong. These contexts, shaped by families' religious, racial, or ethnic identities, often deeply affect parental decision making. We see this in relation to the Navajo communities treated by Maureen Schwarz, where long-standing tensions between the Navajo and white "foreigners" (*bilaganna*) can lead parents to oppose specific, lifesaving medical procedures for their child. It appears again in the case of Muslim parents. As Zahra Ayubi points out, religiously sanctioned gender roles can sometimes render mothers invisible, as male authorities within and outside of the family control the decision process. A leading example of the importance of taking context into account is the case of the African American families discussed by Patrick Smith. Black children are highly and disproportionately represented in the population of low-birth-weight (LBW) and very-low-birth-weight (VLBW) infants who present in many American NICUs. Given the relatively lower economic status of many black families and the existence of other sources of family disruption, NICU caregivers may be led to assume that the presence of these infants in the NICU is a result of economic factors or, worse, personal conduct of the mother such as drug or alcohol abuse. But Smith urges us to look away from such presumptions and pay attention to the unethical and dehumanizing "causes of the causes," which he identifies as systematic racism. Cross-cultural studies show that this demonstrably worsens the health of black women in this country. If we add to this observation the history of black Americans' justifiable mistrust of the medical establishment, we can begin to see how important it is for NICU caregivers to "center at the margins." By this, Smith means that caregivers must shift away from white experience to understand the environments from which their tiny patients emerge and to which they are likely to be returned.

The sixth and final insight for NICU caregivers suggested by these chapters is that despite their many commonalities, religions do not all say the same thing. For example, ritual observances can differ significantly, and, whenever possible, caregivers must be sensitive to this. While mainstream Protestants celebrate baptism as an acknowledgment of the child's value, Mennonites and many other evangelicals explicitly reject infant baptism, and their ritual needs take a different form. Subtle theological differences can attain importance. Gerald Winslow informs us that Adventists do not believe that at death a disembodied soul goes to heaven. Rather, the deceased enters a time of "rest," awaiting the general resurrection. Because of this, says Winslow, "it is not helpful to suggest to Adventists that a deceased loved one is now looking down from heaven."[23] What can be extremely comforting in one case may be disquieting or offensive in another.

Of course, NICU professionals cannot be expected to be experts on all the nuances of the wide variety of religious traditions, but they should always be sensitive to the role of religion in many parents' thinking and decision making. When dealing with parents and families for whom religion is important, NICU caregivers should try to call on the expertise of others. These include hospital chaplains or community-based Protestant pastors, Jewish rabbis, Catholic priests, Muslim imams, Buddhist monks, Hindu pandits, or Native American traditional teachers. When significant numbers of adherents to one or another tradition are represented among parents of the patient population, NICU staff should strive to build relationships with such specialists.

Finally, NICU professionals should also strive to try to become "religious generalists," developing a basic understanding of the beliefs, values, and practices of all those cooperating in the care of newborns. In addition to parents, this includes NICU staff, many of whom bring their own religious commitments to their work. This book is a beginning contribution to the education of parents, families, and NICU caregivers about the importance of religion in the context of family-centered care.

Notes

1. A. J. London, "The Maltese Conjoined Twins. Two Views of Their Separation" and "The Maltese Conjoined Twins. A Separate Peace," *Hastings Center Report* 31, no. 1 (January–February 2001): 48–50; P. Mallia, "Maltese Conjoined Twins," *Hastings Center Report* 31, no. 6 (November–December 2001): 4; D. Wechter, "The Maltese Twins Case," *National Catholic Bioethics Quarterly* 1, no. 4 (Winter 2001): 485; M. C. Kaveny, "Conjoined Twins and Catholic Moral Analysis: Extraordinary Means and Casuistical Consistency," *Kennedy Institute of Ethics Journal* 12, no. 2 (June 2002): 115–40; C. Dyer, "Law, Ethics, and Emotion: The Charlie Gard Case," *BMJ* (July 4, 2017), accessed December 14, 2017, http://www.bmj.com/content/358/bmj.j3152/rr-1; D. Wilkinson and J. Savulescu, "Hard Lessons: Learning from the Charlie Gard Case," *Journal of Medical Ethics*, published online August 2, 2017, accessed December 14, 2017, http://jme.bmj.com/content/early/2017/08/28/medethics-2017-104492.long; A. Caplan and K. M. Folkers, "Charlie Gard and the Limits of Parental Authority," *Hastings Center Report* 47, no. 5 (September 2017): 15–16; J. D. Lantos, "The Tragic Case of Charlie Gard," *JAMA Pediatrics* 171, no. 10 (October 2017): 935–36; A. Gallagher, "What Can We Learn from the Case of Charlie Gard? Perspectives from an Inter-disciplinary Panel Discussion," *Nursing Ethics* 24, no. 7 (November 2017): 775–77; J. J. Paris et al., "The Charlie Gard Case: British and American Approaches to Court Resolution of Disputes over Medical Decisions," *Journal of Perinatology* 37 (2017): 1268–71.

2. Krishnadev Calamur, "Charlie Gard's Parents End Their Fight to Keep Their Child Alive," *The Atlantic*, July 24, 2017, accessed December 14, 2017, https://www.theatlantic.com/news/archive/2017/07/charlie-gard-parents-end-legal-fight/534657/.

3. Helen Harrison, "The Principles for Family-Centered Neonatal Care," *Pediatrics* 92, no. 5 (1993): 643–50.

4. Tracy A. Balboni et al., "Religiousness and Spiritual Support among Advanced Cancer Patients and Associations with End-of-Life Treatment Preferences and Quality of Life," *Journal of Clinical Oncology* 25, no. 5 (2000): 555–59.

5. H. S. Lam et al., "Attitudes toward Treatment of Preterm Infants with a High Risk of Developing Long-term Disabilities," *Pediatrics* 123 (2009): 1501–08.

6. Janet Green, "Living in Hope and Desperate for a Miracle: NICU Nurses Perceptions of Parental Anguish," *Journal of Religion and Health* 54 (2015): 731–44.

7. An exception is the discussion by J. McGuirl and D. Campbell, "Understanding the Role of Religious Views in the Discussion about Resuscitation at the Threshold of Viability," *Journal of Perinatology* 36 (2016): 694–98.

8. Program description available online. Accessed January 6, 2017, https://cmetracker.net/USF/Files/Brochures/342164.pdf.

9. *Religion and Ethics in the Neonatal Intensive Care Unit*, pp. 39–40.

10. Ibid., p. 106.

11. Ibid., p. 239.

12. Ibid., p. 124.

13. bid., pp. 172–174.

14. Christopher Tollefsen, ed., *Artificial Nutrition and Hydration: The New Catholic Debate* (Dordrecht: Springer, 2010).

15. H. Roberts and R. Mitchell, "The Use of Anti-D Prophylaxis in the Management of Miscarriage in General Practice," *Health Bulletin* (Edinburgh) 49, no. 4 (1991): 245–49.

16. *Religion and Ethics in the Neonatal Intensive Care Unit*, p. 118.

17. Ibid., p. 200.

18. Ibid., p. 90.

19. Ibid., p. 41.

20. Ibid., p. 207.

21. Ibid., p. 72.

22. Michael J. Balboni et al., "'It Depends': Viewpoints of Patients, Physicians, and Nurses on Patient-Practitioner Prayer in the Setting of Advanced Cancer," *Journal of Pain Symptom Management* 41, no. 5 (2011): 836–47.

23. *Religion and Ethics in the Neonatal Intensive Care Unit*, p. 222.

1

Judaism and Neonatology

Elliot N. Dorff

Two introductory comments will help readers understand the role and methodology of this essay. First, why might one be interested in Judaism's approach to neonatology? What, if anything, is wrong with the secular American approach?

The answer is that there is nothing wrong with the secular American approach, but it is rooted in a very specific perspective—namely, that of Western liberalism—and Judaism has a different lens on the world. In fact, each of the religions of the world and each of the secular philosophies of the world (e.g., communism, existentialism, liberalism) provides a particular lens of its own. Each religion and philosophy articulates a broad picture of who we are as individuals and as members of a community, and what kind of individual and community we should strive to be. Even though every religion and philosophy portrays human beings, the visions of who we are and who we ought to be are remarkably different.

The American version of Western liberalism was well summarized by Thomas Jefferson in the Declaration of Independence, borrowing from John Locke's work one hundred years earlier. According to that document, it is "self-evident" that we are individuals with rights, including life, liberty, and the pursuit of happiness. As a result, personal autonomy is the gold standard of American medical ethics. As the *Nancy Cruzan* decision of the US Supreme Court asserted in 1990, adults have a right to refuse all medical interventions, including artificial nutrition and hydration. (The reverse is not true: Americans do not have the right to get any medical intervention they want.) So, in end-of-life care generally, it is the patient's wishes that matter, and in medical decisions about neonates, the parents' decisions are legally authoritative—at least within some bounds.[1]

The central story in Judaism, however, is the Exodus from Egypt and the trek to Mount Sinai and then the Promised Land. We leave Egypt not as individuals but as a community. At Sinai, we get not a single right; we get instead 613 commandments. Sometimes rights and duties are reciprocal, but if you get up in the morning under the assumption that you are an individual with rights, then the world owes you; if, on the other hand, you get up with the understanding that you are part of a community with duties, then you owe the world. This is the basis for the strong Jewish commitment to *tikkun olam,* repairing the world, in all areas of life—relieving poverty, fostering education, building conditions for peace, and helping the sick, among others. So, while Jews may be interested in a Jewish perspective on medical matters because it is part of their tradition, both Jews and others may be interested in it because of the unique perspective it has on many issues and what one can learn from it, even if only to see one's own contrasting perspective better.

Gaining Moral Guidance from a Tradition

The second introductory comment that I want to make is this: medicine has advanced significantly in the past fifty years, with neonatology being a prime example. The US Supreme Court in its 1973 *Roe v. Wade* decision maintained that fetal viability occurred only during the third trimester of gestation. Now, children born as early as twenty-three weeks have been kept alive, and even though we know that significant development of the brain and lungs occurs in the last weeks of pregnancy, a child born at thirty-two weeks or later has a very good chance of living a normal life without major deficits.

This, however, raises the Kantian question. The eighteenth-century philosopher Immanuel Kant pointed out that "ought implies can"[2]—that is, that one can be held morally responsible for something only if one can follow the moral norm. It follows from this, conversely, that when one cannot do something, one need not ask whether one should because, after all, there is nothing that can be done. If, however, one can do something, then one must ask whether one should, for there are many things that one can do that one should not. One can, for example, smoke cigarettes, but given what we know about the harms involved, one should not. Now that we can keep very premature infants alive, we must ask whether we should, a question our parents never had to face. That is, the advances of medicine, as wonderful as they are, have made the moral issues surrounding medicine all the more acute.

When we turn to our traditions—whether secular or religious—to give us moral guidance about these matters, however, we face a major methodological problem. The people who created both secular philosophy and the world's religious traditions had no clue about modern medical abilities. As a result, no philosophical, legal, or religious tradition even contemplated people having these abilities, let alone provided guidance in how to use them. How, then, should we use our traditions to gain moral guidance from them?

One approach is to say that if a tradition says nothing on point about a given topic, then we should look elsewhere for moral guidance. The advantage of this approach is that it is honest: Jewish traditional texts and practices have nothing to say about whether to save a severely compromised, premature infant because until recently that infant could not be saved. The disadvantages of this approach, however, are major. It is not only Judaism that has no experience with these questions; every other philosophy, legal system, and religion is in the same boat. So, where should one turn for moral instruction on these new issues in neonatology? Furthermore, if we say that Judaism is irrelevant to all matters on which it lacks specific instruction, then it will turn out to be irrelevant to a large proportion of life, for many, many things have changed since the classical texts—and even the medieval and modern ones—were written. One of the things that Jews expect their tradition to give them, though, is moral guidance, so this method will be bad for both Judaism and Jews.

The opposite end of the spectrum is to say that by hook or by crook, we will find something in the tradition that can be interpreted to apply to new circumstances. The advantage of this approach is that the interpretation provides a link to the tradition, however tenuous, and this reinforces one's sense that the tradition is worthwhile. It also makes the tradition relevant to everything. The disadvantages, however, are serious, for it often entails doing eisegesis rather than exegesis— that is, it involves reading what one wants into the tradition rather than discovering what the tradition is saying by interpreting it reasonably. Especially if one is grounded in the Jewish tradition, which has a very sophisticated sense of the multiple ways in which any given text can be interpreted (the Rabbis say that "There are seventy faces to the Torah," seventy being just a big number[3]), the line between proper interpretation and improperly making the text mean whatever you want it to mean is often both thin and not clear. Nevertheless, when you find yourself making a text mean what you know is not the actual meaning of the text or even a reasonable extension of it, you are no longer gaining guidance from tradition, and you are deceiving yourself and misrepresenting the tradition if you think you are.

How should we gain moral guidance from our tradition on matters that it does not contemplate, let alone deal with? I would suggest a middle ground between these two extremes. Specifically, when our tradition does say something relevant to the question at hand—and we will see later that classical Jewish texts do say some important things about the status of the fetus and neonate—then we should certainly engage with those texts. We must, however, understand them in their historical contexts. Sometimes a text will accurately reflect what we know to be true according to modern science, but sometimes the science of times past is very different from what we know now. Thus, in using relevant texts from the tradition, we must evaluate which to use and how to use them.

When there are no texts or traditions relevant to the question at hand, how-ever, we should do what I call "depth theology." That is, we should identify the underlying beliefs and practices of the tradition that bear on this case and apply them to it. People within the tradition may well disagree on how best to do that, especially because by hypothesis we are talking about a case in which there are no precedents on point. For that matter, people might disagree about how to apply a text even when it is directly on point! So, one must expect and even be thankful for the varying approaches that those within a tradition take, based on the varying lines they draw back to elements of the tradition. To use this method, though, one has to tolerate a lot of argument and very little certainty—a very familiar and comfortable place for Jews who inherit a feisty tradition in which Abraham, Moses, Isaiah, and Job, among others, argued with God and in which every page of the Talmud is one argument after another!

The role of rabbis in advising parents of neonates will clearly vary, depending on which of the previous approaches one takes. This can be seen most graph-ically in the advance directives for health care that each of the modern movements in Judaism has formulated. The Orthodox version simply states that the person wants to abide by Jewish law in his or her end-of-life care and then lists the rabbi whom his or her doctors should consult. On the other end of the spectrum, the Reform advance directive included in Rabbi Richard Address's 1995 book, *A Time to Prepare*, in accordance with the Reform emphasis on per-sonal autonomy, provides a grid to indicate one's choices. Down the side is a list of possible medical interventions, and across the top are four categories: I want; I want treatment tried, but if no clear improvement, stop; I am undecided; I do not want. The Conservative advance directive, reflecting the Conservative Movement's commitment to Jewish law, lists ten common scenarios at the end of life that require decisions and then lists the decisions that are conso-nant with Jewish law as interpreted by the two rabbinic rulings approved by the Conservative Movement's Committee on Jewish Law and Standards (CJLS), with the decisions approved by both rulings in block print and those approved by only one of them in italics. This, then, indicates not only the importance of Jewish law in making such decisions but also the role of the individual pa-tient in deciding which of several approved options to take.[4] Thus, rabbis in the Orthodox community, at least in theory, decide the course of medical care for their constituents; rabbis in the Reform movement serve as consultants along with doctors and others the patient might choose to ask in making his or her own decision; and rabbis in the Conservative movement serve as educators in Jewish law so that the patient or his or her parents make a decision in conso-nance with it as well as ministering to the specific needs of the patient or, in the case of a neonate, his or her parents.

The Moral and Legal Status of the Neonate

The Jewish tradition's position on the status of the neonate begins with this passage in the Torah:

> When men fight, and one of them pushes a pregnant woman and a miscarriage results, but no other damage ensues, the one responsible shall be fined according as the woman's husband may exact from him, the payment to be based on reckoning. But if other damage ensues, the penalty shall be life for life, eye for eye, tooth for tooth, hand for hand, foot for foot, burn for burn, wound for wound, bruise for bruise.[5]

Even though the Rabbis later changed "eye for eye" to monetary compensation,[6] the fact that the Torah imposes only monetary compensation for the fetus and the harsher penalty of an eye for an eye for injury to the woman indicates that the status of the fetus is less than that of a full-fledged human being like the mother. From this, the Rabbis of the Mishnah, the first compilation of the classical Rabbis' legal decisions and ethical values (edited c. 200 C.E.), deduce that, in their time, when cesarean deliveries were almost definitely lethal for the mother, if a woman was having difficulty in childbirth and both the fetus and the mother could not be saved, we must dismember the fetus within her so that she would live:

> If a woman has [life-threatening] difficulty in childbirth, one dismembers the embryo in her, limb by limb, because her life takes precedence over its life. Once its greater part [some versions: "head"] has emerged, it may not be touched, for we do not set aside one life for another.[7]

Although this Mishnah's primary concern is to proclaim that we should save the life of the woman in childbirth even at the expense of the life of the fetus, it also defines when the fetus becomes a neonate with the full legal status of any other human being—namely, at birth. In practice, this means that if the baby's head (in a typical birth) or greater part (in a breech birth) had emerged and the doctors still could not extract the baby from the mother, then, assuming they could not save both, they would save whichever one they had the better chance of saving, which is the usual triage rule later in life as well.

The Rabbis of the Talmud were medically incorrect in something else they say about neonates. Specifically, they believed that a fetus born at seven months would survive, but one born at eight months would not.[8] We now know that the longer the fetus is in the mother's womb, the better, for even in the last weeks of pregnancy, the fetus' brain and lungs develop.[9] That mistake, however, does not affect how later Jewish commentators understand the proper care of the fetus once born, for then, as the Mishnah cited previously attests and as most contemporary rabbis assert,[10] it is a full-fledged human being worthy of the same kind of medical care that we would give older children or adults. So, we now need to step back to consider some underlying Jewish convictions that define how Judaism understands health care in general, disabilities, and end-of-life care.[11]

Fundamental Jewish Convictions that Set the Context for the Care of Neonates

1. *Medicine.* Although the Bible says in a number of places that God inflicts illness (usually connected with sin) and brings healing,[12] the Jewish tradition did not interpret those passages to mean that human beings should refrain from interfering with God's prerogatives. That is because another passage from Exodus 21 asserts that when two men are fighting, the assailant "must surely heal" the injured party, from which the Rabbis deduce that it is at least permissible to engage in medical care.[13] From the commandment in Deuteronomy 22 that requires a finder of a lost object to return it, the Rabbis deduced that we have not only permission to seek to heal but also a duty to do so, for people usually do and should value their health more than any object they own.[14] Finally, based on Leviticus 19:16 ("You should not stand idly by your brother") or Leviticus 19:18 ("Love your neighbor as yourself"), the Rabbis rule that the duty to seek to heal applies not only to the physician, who has special training, but also to the whole community.[15] So, the doctor is not an intruder on God's role in sickness and health, but rather is the agent and partner of God in helping people avoid, cure, and ameliorate disease.

This view of the doctor's role will explain why there has been a virtual love affair between Judaism and medicine for the past two thousand years. During that time, in fact, many rabbis were also trained and served as physicians, Maimonides perhaps the most famous among them. (The much longer time it takes to educate a physician nowadays has made that combination of professions rare.) This attitude toward physicians and medicine also explains why Jews tend to be very aggressive in the use of medical care.

2. *The disabled.* At the same time, another Jewish conviction plays an important role in how Judaism approaches neonatal care—namely, its understanding of disabilities. The Torah asserts in its very first chapter that the human being is created in the image of God.[16] Exactly what aspect of the human being is divine is a matter of dispute in later Jewish sources. Maimonides thinks that it is the human intellect; some think that God and humans share a spiritual nature; but

the Garden of Eden story makes it seem that it is the ability of humans to distinguish right from wrong and to act on that basis that is the divine element in human beings. Whatever it is, the image of God is still evident in a person who has committed a capital crime, for Deuteronomy 21:22–23 asserts that even such a person must be taken down from the execution post before nightfall "because it is a curse of God" for any human being to hang overnight in that position.

Disabled people clearly share in this image of God, whatever their disability. In fact, we all have strengths and weaknesses, and many in the disabled community call those of us who do not have a clear disability "the temporarily abled." That should give each of us pause, and it should motivate us to respect and take care of the disabled. Furthermore, precisely because people seeing a disabled person might have an immediate, negative aesthetic reaction or silently say to themselves, "Thank God I am not like that," the Jewish tradition instructs us that, upon seeing a disabled person, one is supposed to recite this blessing: "Praised are You, Lord, Sovereign of the universe, who has made people different." The blessing is a liturgical way of educating us emotionally to appreciate the ultimate worth of people, regardless of their disabilities.[17]

This has important implications for how we think of intervening medically with neonates. On one hand, we need to do whatever we can to change or at least alleviate any deficits they have; on the other, people are to be appreciated as being created in the image of God no matter what the level of their abilities or disabilities may be. This does not necessarily mean that we must "pull out all the stops" in trying to save every prematurely born child, as we will see in the next few paragraphs, but it does mean that the decision not to do so cannot be based on an assessment that the child will not be normal.

3. *People are mortal.* Balancing the aggressive attitude toward the use of medicine in Judaism is the realization that we are mortal. This is expressed as early as the Garden of Eden story, in which Adam and Eve were able to eat of the fruit of the tree of the knowledge of good and evil but not of the tree of life,[18] which is a mythic way of acknowledging that people can distinguish good from bad and act on the basis of that knowledge, but we do not live forever. Later, Ecclesiastes asserts, "There is a time to be born and a time to die."[19]

Until recently in human history, doctors could do little to reverse the dying process. That was certainly true in the era before vaccines and antibiotics, and consequently there is little in the Jewish tradition that gives us guidance about deciding when to intervene and how. The *Shulhan Arukh*, an important sixteenth-century code of Jewish law, asserts that we may not hasten the dying process, but Rabbi Moses Isserles, who wrote a gloss on the code, says that, on the other hand, we should not prolong the dying process either.[20] Until recently, that provided a bright red line as to what was acceptable and what was not. The advances of medicine have made that line harder to discern, however, and that is especially true with regard to neonates, where it often is not clear whether our interventions are just postponing the inevitable or are providing a child with a lease on life. This is the Kantian question discussed earlier in its morally excruciating form.

This is a problem not only for the physicians and nurses involved but also for the parents. Before the late 1960s, if a child was born prematurely and could not be saved, doctors would take the infant into another room and let him or her die, and they would tell the mother, who was under anesthesia during the birth, and the father, who was in the waiting room, that the child was born dead. The parents were thus spared the agonizing decision of whether to ask the physicians to do their best to keep the child alive or to ask them to keep the child comfortable as he or she died. It also saved insurance companies and the government large expenditures of money in trying to keep alive children who may or may not live and, if so, who may have significant deficits and would need frequent and costly interventions throughout their life.

However, with the advent of the Lamaze method of childbirth in the late 1960s, in which the mother is awake during childbirth and the father is at her side, the parents would see the birth of their child, and that imposed on them the difficult decision of how to proceed when the child was born prematurely or with major deficits. They also needed to factor in how they would pay for the child's special care, often throughout his or her life, and the effects that caring for this child would have on their other children and on their marriage. (Many couples divorce under the psychological and financial pressures of caring for a child with special needs.) Doctors advising such parents would also have to take into account the morally and sometimes medically murky questions of the chances of saving the child, the future health status of the child, and the money involved in caring for him or her, should they decide to try to save the child's life.

This question, though, applies to older people as well, and contemporary Jewish moral and legal discussions of end-of-life care are much more developed than Jewish discussions of neonates, so it is worthwhile to summarize that discussion here. In an instance of the methodological problem I discussed earlier, because there are only four sources in the entire Jewish tradition that even contemplate that humans would have the ability to prolong the life of someone who was dying, and even those sources are far removed from the medical realities of today, it is not surprising that contemporary rabbis disagree about what should be done when people have terminal illnesses.

Some, such as Rabbi J. David Bleich, a professor at Yeshiva University (Orthodox), maintain that one must do all that one can to keep the person alive, even if the person is comatose or severely compromised in other ways, for "every moment of life is of infinite value" and no considerations of quality of life may be entertained.[21] The official position of the Modern Orthodox organization of rabbis, the Rabbinical Council of America, asserts that one may withhold machines and medications but not withdraw them once applied.[22] Rabbi Eliezer Waldenberg in Israel, however, suggests putting the machines supporting a patient on a timer so that the timer can turn off the machine if the physician determines that it is not helping the patient to recover.[23] All Orthodox writers maintain that artificial nutrition and hydration must be supplied if the person cannot eat, but there is a dispute among Orthodox authorities as to whether to accept the whole-brain death criterion for determining death or to insist on the traditional criteria of cessation of breath and heartbeat.[24]

Rabbi Avram Reisner (Conservative) interprets Jewish law to say that machines and medications may be both withheld and withdrawn because they are interventions that not everybody needs to live, but artificial nutrition and hydration must be administered and may not be removed until the person dies because everyone needs food and liquids.[25] On the other hand, in another ruling endorsed by the Conservative Movement's Committee on Jewish Law and Standards along with that of Rabbi Reisner, I maintain that machines, medications, and artificial nutrition and hydration may be withheld or withdrawn because I see artificial nutrition and hydration as medicine rather than as food, given that it comes into the body differently from how we normally eat and drink and it lacks many of the traits that we normally associate with food and liquids, in which there are differences in taste, temperature, texture, and so forth. The criterion of whether to maintain life support or not is in my view the welfare of the patient, as determined by his or her own directives, either in person or, if he or she is unconscious or otherwise mentally incompetent, in an advance directive, if the patient created one, or by the surrogate decision maker's knowledge of the patient.[26]

The same dispute of whether artificial nutrition and hydration may or should be removed from a terminally ill patient exists in Reform rabbinic rulings.[27] Thus, to varying degrees, rabbis writing in our own day across the full spectrum of Jewish ideologies permit what some call "passive euthanasia."

That is not true, however, for what writers variously call "active euthanasia" (drugs of a lethal dose or other means to hasten death, administered by someone other than the patient), "assisted suicide" (administered by the patient with the help of the physician or someone else), or "aid in dying" (which is the new, less judgmental term used for assisted suicide), all of which are disparaged by rabbis of all the Jewish movements. Some of that opposition comes directly from the distinction in classical Jewish law mentioned previously—that we should not delay the dying process, but we should not hasten it either. Others adduce additional reasons to oppose active measures to bring about the person's death, including these: (1) our bodies belong to God, not to us humans, and thus we do not have the right to destroy them; (2) if we allow assisted suicide, insurance companies, including governmental ones like Medicare and Medicaid, will be all too willing to subsidize that shorter and less expensive path to death and will refuse to pay for the long-term care of those who refuse to take that path—in other words, "may" commit suicide will quickly become "financially must"; and (3) money complicates the situation in other ways as well, so the motives for asking for assisted suicide on the part of the patient ("I do not want to squander the assets I want to leave to my children") or the children ("We want Mom to die in a relatively short time so that she does not waste money on her futile care— money that would otherwise come to us ") are not always as pure as they are made out to be—namely, we only want Mom's pain to stop; and (4) often requests for assistance in dying derive from a patient's depression, but then the proper response to treat the depression is through visits of family and friends and, if necessary, medications—not to assist the person to die.[28]

By and large, the same approach to caring for adults at the end of life applies to neonates as well. That is, if the parents, with the advice of their physicians, decide that it would not be in the interests of the child to sustain his or her life due to extensive deficits, then the parents have the right to ask the doctors to let nature take its course while keeping the child comfortable. If, on the other hand, the parents, again with the advice of their doctors, decide that the child has a decent chance to live a meaningful life, they have the right to ask the physicians to try to make that possible.

Although most rabbis writing about these matters treat the care of neonates in the same way they approach the care of adults whose health is severely compromised, some do not. For example, Rabbi Avram Reisner has written a rabbinic ruling that was approved unanimously by the Conservative Movement's CJLS, with this conclusion:

1. Abortion of the fetus is permitted throughout pregnancy for cause.
2. The claim of the potential life of the fetus to our ministrations is greater upon attaining viability, that is, after seven months (31–32 weeks by obstetrical count).
3. Ordinarily, newborns must be cared for as we would care for any adult.
4. Severely deformed and compromised newborns are classed as born dying, and treatments aimed at their survival may be discontinued. Severe deformity refers to anencephaly, trisomies 13 and 18, or other similar large scale genetic deformities. Jewish law does not insist on aggressive treatment in such cases. The term does not apply to lesser deformities, such as trisomy 21 (Down's syndrome).
5. Prematurity is generally to be considered part of the category of lesser deformities. In cases of severe prematurity, the rabbi, in consultation with the family and physician, may conclude that the infant should be classed as unable to survive, and so even though he interprets Jewish law to require

the use of artificial nutrition and hydration for adults, he would not require that for neonates.

6. In fact, everything said here is said as guidance to the rabbi who must carefully assess the case in consultation with the family and physicians in order to determine the proper course in the instant case.[29]

Similarly, in the Reconstructionist Movement, a theory and practice of Judaism that is based on Rabbi Mordecai Kaplan's interpretation of Judaism as "an evolving, religious civilization" and that originally was the left wing of the Conservative movement but became in 1968 a small, independent movement with its own seminary and synagogues, Rabbi David Teutsch has written this:

Occasionally a baby is born with such severe medical problems that the chances of survival without constant medical intervention are negligible, and the infant's future is likely to be one of constant pain. In such a case, withholding or withdrawing extraordinary medical measures that would preserve the infant's life is the merciful, though tragic, thing to do. That is in the parents' interest and in the community interest, and is *l'tovato*, in the infant's interest. This approach can be applied in the days following birth as medical facts become known; however, after 30 days the infant is seen as a fully viable person who must be treated in a way aimed at sustaining the infant's well-being. One must weigh the benefit of invasive treatments against comfort measures to determine the infant's best interest.[30]

On the other hand, in the Orthodox world, with some exceptions, the same aggressive treatment that is required for older people to keep them alive, regardless of the quality of their life, is required also with regard to neonates. Rabbi Avraham Steinberg, MD, is typical in asserting this:

It is forbidden to *hasten the death* of a premature or handicapped baby, such as by starvation, even if it can live only for a short time. Even if it is suffering, one must treat it as best as possible and not hasten its death. The parents must do everything possible to treat their handicapped newborn. Even if the parents refuse lifesaving surgery, it should be done against their wishes and they can be held responsible for the expenses. Coercion, however, is not necessary for purely elective surgery to improve the baby's status, for example, so that it can live at home rather than be institutionalized.

Desertion or abandonment of a newborn, for whatever reason, is totally against Jewish tradition and Jewish law. Never in Jewish sources has such an occurrence been described. Rather, in spite of pain and anguish, Jewish parents take and raise their handicapped children.[31]

So, there is a spectrum of positions regarding newborns with a definitely limited future and likely death in infancy, such as Trisomy 13 or 18, Tay-Sachs disease, or Lesch-Nyhan syndrome, with Orthodox rabbis maintaining that everything must be done to keep the baby alive, Conservative rabbis allowing for less aggressive treatment in such cases than would be appropriate for older children or adults, and Reconstructionist and Reform rabbis leaving the decision to the parents but advising that the child should be kept comfortable but treated with the goal of letting nature take its course without medical interference ("palliative" or "hospice" care). Rabbis in all movements would want the child, like all patients, to be kept as comfortable as possible, whether or not medical interventions were being applied in an effort to extend the child's life.[32]

Rabbi Steinberg's last assertion in the previous quotation—that abandonment of a newborn "is totally against Jewish tradition and Jewish law"—is also shared by the other denominations of Judaism. Although such a stand might seem obvious, it has not been obvious to societies historically or even to some today. As Rabbi Steinberg points out, in many ancient and early modern societies, abandonment or even infanticide of defective newborns was the norm. Both Plato[33] and Aristotle[34] recommend it; Plato says that even normal children of socially undesirable parents should be killed. Furthermore, "As recently as the early 1800s in Europe, up to a third of live-born infants were killed or abandoned by their parents."[35] In modern China, female fetuses are often aborted (or, until the government closed this opportunity, carried to term and given up for foreign adoption) because only one child per family is generally allowed, with some exceptions, and there is a cultural preference for boys.[36]

4. *Health care as one of a number of communal obligations.* Who pays for the extensive care necessary to save the child—or whether anyone should bear the moral or legal burden to pay for such procedures if the parents want them to be done—is a difficult social question, one that American society to date has not been willing to answer in any meaningful way. Classical Jewish sources do not even talk about the costs of health care, except to say that men have the duty to provide it for their wives as a condition of marriage[37] and that those who injure others must pay for their victims' medical expenses.[38] Until the middle of the twentieth century, curative health care was usually ineffective and therefore inexpensive, and thus Jewish sources understandably do not directly address the question of how to distribute it when it is costly.

Jewish sources do, however, address how to distribute scarce resources in two other arenas of life—namely, in distributing aid to the poor and in redeeming captives.[39] If we use those sources as a guide, we find that although the Jewish tradition very much appreciates health care and the role of those who provide it, it also requires that communities provide for their other needs, including education, religious services, responsiveness to the needs of the poor, and redemption of captives.[40] These sources would probably construe spending the amounts of money required to sustain severely compromised neonates as fiscally unwise and even irresponsible if the other needs of the community could not then be met.

Furthermore, Jewish authorities are universal in saying that pain must be alleviated. As a result, if the procedure to cure a neonate of his or her ills will cause great pain, especially over a long period of time and maybe even during his or her entire life, that, too, is a factor to be considered in deciding whether or not to engage in such medical interventions.

In addition, the Torah's commandment is to heal (Exodus 21:19), not to extend life per se. Until recently in human history, it was presumed that any extension of life was itself an act of healing and therefore required, and there are still some rabbis who maintain that position. In contemporary times, however, it has become clear that some medical interventions are futile and, worse, amount to battering the patient for no good reason. Thus, most rabbis across the religious spectrum, although in differing degrees, would allow or even recommend that life support be withheld or withdrawn when it is not going to cure the patient. This same risk-to-benefit analysis that applies to older children and to adults applies to neonates as well.

Clearly, these general guidelines need to be honed to determine exactly how much of a given community's resources should be spent on neonatal care. To my knowledge, that has not yet been done in any thorough way. Instead, the amount of money any particular family, insurance company, or government is willing and able to spend on neonatal care depends on their resources and other needs. Jewish law would support that kind of pragmatic reasoning, for it demands, as indicated earlier, that communities attend to the range of their needs, not only to their medical ones.

5. *Parents' obligations to children.* The Jewish tradition defines both children's obligations to their parents and parents' obligations to their children. The Talmud's list of filial obligations includes feeding one's elderly parents when they cannot feed themselves and helping them to get from one place to another when they cannot walk by themselves, but its list of parental duties does not include medical care of any sort. This is not surprising in light of the historical context of this discussion, for until very recently in human history, when a child was born prematurely or with major deficits, there was nothing the parents or doctors could do to maintain the child's life. Even the diseases and infections of older children were largely unpreventable and incurable until various times during the last century. So, while parents clearly have the legal right and duty to make decisions for their children under the age of majority, which Jewish law sets as twelve-and-a-half for girls and thirteen for boys, and while they certainly must act for the welfare of their children in all matters, including medical ones, the classical sources do not spell out specific ways in which parents are required to

care for their children medically—except to teach them to swim![41] With regard to neonates, this means that parents should follow the general Jewish rules about health care described previously.

Visiting the Sick

As we move now from the medical and financial consideration of neonatal care to the emotional and psychological factors in such care, the duty in Jewish law to visit the sick comes into play, for the parents of the neonate will need substantial emotional and even practical support—whether they try to save the baby or not. The choice to try to save the baby will involve long periods of stays in the hospital and frequent emotional ups and downs. As a result, the couple may need care for their older children and even require practical help with grocery shopping and taking care of the house, among other chores. If they choose to let the baby die, they will probably still need practical help for a while and emotional support before the child's death and as they begin the mourning process.

Most of us do not like to visit the sick, especially when they are in hospitals, for reasons that include these:

1. On a physical level, we do not want to catch a disease from the person we visit or any of the other people in the hospital, whether that fear is warranted or not.
2. Even if the ill present no physical danger to us, they remind us of our own vulnerability to illness and even our own mortality, neither of which we like to contemplate. The very smells, sights, and sounds of hospitals make those of us not used to such phenomena feel as if we are in a threatening and strange place.
3. Furthermore, engaging with the sick is often depressing and, in the case of the parents of neonates, sad, for we know they were hoping for a full-term pregnancy and a normal child. Instead, they are dealing with an early birth that has the potential for major deficits in the child and possibly even some difficult medical decisions to determine how aggressively they want the doctors to try to keep the child alive.
4. This then raises yet another question: What do you say to the parents of a neonate who either has severe deficits or who has died? Some remarks are clearly off limits, such as "Better luck next time," or "God must be punishing you." So, at least some of the things that one should *not* say are clear, but what *do* you say? If the child is alive, you do not want to dwell on the topic of his or her precarious situation because that is depressing and scary, but if you do not mention it, it becomes the elephant in the room that

nobody wants to recognize and that everyone dances around. So, what do you say to the parents, and how? The whole situation is uncomfortable for everyone involved.

We moderns are by no means the first to feel this way. Our ancestors did not have to go to hospitals to see ill friends or family members, for until very recently in human history, people endured their illnesses at home. On the other hand, though, the lack of medical knowledge about which diseases are contagious must have made our ancestors fear visiting the sick even more than we do. It is precisely because people often have an aversion to visiting the sick that the Jewish tradition made it a *mitzvah* not just in the sense of a nice thing to do, but in the original sense of that word as a commanded and obligatory act. Jews are therefore duty-bound to visit the sick, whether we want to do so or not.

There are other reasons the tradition supplies, however, to visit the sick. First, the Rabbis assert that in doing so, as in providing for the poor and the bereaved, we imitate God:

> Rabbi Hamma, son of Rabbi Hanina, said: "What is the meaning of the verse, 'Follow the Lord your God' (Deuteronomy 13:5)? Is it possible for a mortal to follow God's Presence? After all, the Torah says, 'For the Lord your God is a consuming fire' (Deuteronomy 4:24). Rather, the verse means to teach us that we should follow the *attributes* of the Holy Blessed One. As God clothes the naked, . . .you should clothe the naked; the Holy Blessed One visited the sick, as it says, 'The Lord appeared to him by the terebinths of Mamre' (Genesis 18:1) [after the account of Abraham's circumcision], so too you should visit the sick. The Holy One buried the dead, . . . so too should you; the Holy One comforted mourners, so too should you."[42]

Second, the tradition understood that *illness is isolating*. People, though, are social beings. Although we need some time to be alone, and although some of us are more gregarious than others, all of us crave company, at least from time to time. That is why the harshest punishment in prison settings, short of execution and torture, is solitary confinement. Thus, it is not surprising that the isolation of illness adds to its ill effects, if not to the illness itself:

> Rabbi Abba son of Rabbi Hanina said: He who visits an invalid takes away a sixtieth of his pain [or, in another version, a sixtieth of his illness]. . . . Rabbi Helbo fell ill. Rabbi Kahana then went [to the house of study] and proclaimed, "Rabbi Helbo is ill." Nobody, however, visited him. Rabbi Kahana rebuked them [the disciples], saying, "Did it ever happen that one of Rabbi Akiba's students fell ill, and the [rest of the] disciples did not visit him?" So Rabbi Akiba himself

entered [Rabbi Helbo's house] to visit him, and because they swept and sprinkled the ground before him [that is, cleaned the house and put it in order], Rabbi Helbo recovered. Rabbi Akiba then went forth and lectured: He who does not visit the sick is like one who sheds blood. When Rabbi Dimi came [from Palestine], he said: He who visits the sick causes him to live, while he who does not causes him to die. How does he cause this? . . . He who visits the sick prays that he may live, . . . [while] he who does not visit the sick prays neither that he may live nor die.[43]

This Talmudic story becomes the basis for later Jewish law:

Visiting the sick is an obligation incumbent on everyone. Even the great [those of high social status] visit the small [those of low social status]. And we should visit many times each day, and all who add visits are to be praised as long as they do not burden [the sick person]. And anyone who visits the sick is as if he took away a part of his illness and made things easier for him; anyone who fails to visit the sick is as if he sheds blood.[44]

What, then, should one do and say while visiting the sick? As I discuss elsewhere,[45] the Jewish tradition has much to tell us about how to visit older children and adults, including advice on whether to sit or stand, what to talk about, and how to support both the patient and his or her family. Because most premature infants in the past died, the Jewish materials on what to say to parents of premature infants comes primarily in the sections on mourning, and some of it, as one might imagine, is heavily influenced by theologically questionable assertions or clear superstitions. So, for example, when I visited a couple I know after their toddler wandered off and drowned in a pool in the backyard of the people they were visiting, the mother told me that her ultra-Orthodox uncle had told her that God imposes tragedies like this only on those who can bear them. She was very angry with him, and she asked me whether I believe that. I said, "No," and I then reminded her of some of the classical Jewish texts we had studied together that call attention to the limits of our knowledge, including our ability to discern why bad things happen to good people.

On some occasions, I have seen people unearth superstitions, including the use of amulets and incantations to ward off evil spirits; on others, people try magic to force God to change the situation. Although I understand that people in distress grasp at straws, the Talmud insists that, "we may not depend on miracles"[46] and, "the world conducts itself according to its usual custom"[47]—that is, the laws of nature work consistently. So, it is *not* a good idea to invoke superstitions or suggest that some miracle may occur that will falsify what the doctors are telling the parents.

What *should* one do when visiting parents of a sick newborn? First, the very fact that you are there is important because it tells the parents that they are not alone in coping with this. Second, see if you can help them with any of the practical necessities of life—buy groceries, carpool their other children, and so forth. Most important, though, is to help them express their fear, anger, bewilderment, and all the other emotions that normally accompany the premature birth of a child. Do not say, "I know what you must be feeling" unless you, too, have had a sick newborn, and even then these parents may react differently from the way you did. Instead of imposing your own thoughts and feelings on the parents, ask them to express theirs. You should not ask something general, like, "How do you feel?" because the answer to that is obvious—scared and angry. Ask instead something specific, like, "What did the doctors say?" and then ask how they are responding to that prognosis. *Do not* offer advice about how to treat the child medically; that is the doctor's job. Also, do not forget to hug the parents when they need that kind of physical demonstration of support.

What if the neonate has died? One of the problems facing parents who have lost a newborn is others' inattention to the depth and degree of their loss, especially if the child was severely compromised from the start. Thus, such parents often feel doubly isolated—in their loss, and in the lack of appreciation of their loss.[48]

To avoid exacerbating the pain of the loss of a neonate, it is critical that visitors refrain from judging the depth of the parents' pain. Just because the neonate lived a very short life or lacked many of the faculties that enable people to live so that imminent death was expected does not mean that the parents need to mourn any less than they would a child who had lived for a while. Yes, parents who mourn a child who died after years of life have many memories, as do all other family members and friends who knew the child, and parents of a neonate who died shortly after birth do not have those memories. They must, though, mourn their fantasies of their life with their child that every couple has while the woman is pregnant as well as face the new, sad reality that their lives will continue without the child and the hole that that leaves in their lives. Moreover, they had virtually no time at all to enjoy this new addition to their family. So, their grief is different from that of parents who lose a child after months or years, but it is no less painful. In any case, visitors should not be comparing depths of sadness in the various situations that bring them to support grieving parents; they should instead acknowledge the loss and the pain that losing a child brings, hug the parents, and support them emotionally and practically in any way they can.

Mourning Rites

If people understand and act on the need to visit the ill, they even more readily recognize that friends and family members who have lost a loved one need to have others surrounding them at that time to help them cope with their loss. This is especially true if the loss is sudden, unexpected, and tragic, as it often is in the case of premature infants; but it is also true if the deceased suffered through an illness for a long time, such that death was ultimately a blessing for everyone, including (perhaps especially) the deceased. After all, every death is a loss, and relatives and friends need help in making their peace with it. Even more important, they need others to help them mourn.

Some forms of aid that mourners need are material and easy to recognize. Thus, Jewish tradition mandates that people bring food with them so that the mourning family does not have to worry about such matters during the seven days of mourning (*shiva*). Coordinating who is bringing what and making sure that people are there to set the food out on the table and clean up afterward are essential parts of this duty, and those who perform these tasks are doing a real, concrete service for the mourners. Similarly, helping the family with carpool duty for their children and other mundane but essential tasks in life are doing a real service. Finally, showing up for a *minyan* (prayer quorum) during each morning and evening of the *shiva* period and walking the mourners around the block after the last morning service of the week to symbolize their reentry into life are clear, physical things that one can and should do.

The emotionally harder part of fulfilling one's duty during *shiva* is to help the bereaved mourn. What does it mean to mourn, and how can one help? Mourning is the process by which relatives and friends separate themselves first physically and then psychologically from the deceased. We separate ourselves physically from the person who has died through the funeral and burial. To make that separation clear to everyone attending a Jewish funeral, it is customary for everyone at the interment to shovel three shovels-full of earth onto the casket once it has been lowered into the ground. The thud the dirt makes as it hits the casket makes it clear to everyone in a very graphic way that the deceased will no longer be part of our physical world.

That, though, only begins the process of separating ourselves from the deceased psychologically. To do that, everyone who knew him or her—and especially close relatives and friends—must express (literally, "press out of themselves") their memories of the deceased. People do that by talking out their memories, crying as they think of some of them and laughing as they think of others. That is true for adults and even children who have lived a number of years, and elsewhere I describe how people can help family and friends engage in that process effectively and without embarrassment.[49]

What, though, are the Jewish rites with regard to a newborn who has died? The *Shulhan Arukh*, an important sixteenth-century code of Jewish law, says this:

> For a child regarding whom we do not know for certain that its months of pregnancy were complete, who died within thirty (days of birth) or even on the thirtieth day, we do not rend [our clothes in mourning or perform any of the other mourning rites].[50]

Picking up on the conditional clause of this ruling, a later commentator says that when we know for certain that a child's months of gestation were complete, we must rend garments and observe full mourning rites. This is based on the comment of the Mishnah that, "A boy one day old counts to his father, his mother, and all his relatives as if he were a fully grown man."[51] The Talmud interprets this to refer to mourning when it is established that the months of the baby's gestation were fully completed.[52] According to later Jewish law, the parents should, as is customary in mourning, rend their clothes and observe the seven days of full mourning and the thirty days of partial mourning, including the recitation of a prayer traditionally said by mourners, the *mourner's kaddish*. If the child died within thirty days of birth, no other public rites are practiced, there is no eulogy, and it is only the family and not the public who participate in the rites of mourning.[53] Only if the baby died more than thirty days after its birth are full mourning rites observed, not only by the family but also by the community.[54]

Modern medicine has given us increased ability to determine the gestational age of a neonate, and according to some authorities, this should affect how we mourn a neonate. Even within the Conservative Movement, there is a range of opinions, all validated as within traditional bounds by its Committee on Jewish Law and Standards (CJLS).

Rabbi Isodoro Aizenberg, in his 1987 ruling, asserted that, "If the baby was born prematurely and died before 30 days are over, the baby should be treated as a [miscarried] fetus. In this case, there is burial, but no other mourning rituals are practiced."[55] In contrast, Rabbi Stephanie Dickstein, in her 1992 ruling, says this:

Premature Infants
. . . Since a majority of the infants born alive after twenty-seven weeks of gestation can be expected to survive, we are no longer dealing with the same situation as our predecessors did. For them, premature birth meant that the infant's chance of survival beyond the first few days of life was doubtful. The intention of the halakhah [Jewish law] in taking advantage of the principal of leniency in

a case of doubt, so that it distinguished between the death of a premature infant and one who was full term, was to avoid burdening parents repeatedly with the regulation periods of mourning.

Today, we have a different reality. A majority of the infants born alive, even after a gestational period of only twenty-seven weeks, can be expected to survive. By that point in the pregnancy, most parents expect to bring a baby home from the hospital, even if it requires technical assistance at the beginning of its life. When we do not require mourning for an infant who dies after that time, we are not being sensitive to the parents. Our insensitivity contrasts with the sensitivity which we assume on the part of the Rabbis when, confronted by high rates of infant mortality, they sought to avoid burdening the parents. Under present medical conditions, we can no longer justify the leniency of not requiring the parents of a premature infant who dies to observe the rites of mourning as already described above.

Between Premature and Not Gestationally Viable

How premature is too premature, too uncertain, for us to require mourning? This is one point on which I feel that both the CJLS as a Movement-wide halakhic authority, and individual rabbis, must retain some flexibility. The boundaries of medicine's ability to save the lives of tiny infants are constantly being pushed back. Certainly, our limit should not go back beyond the five months at which we begin to require burial. However, between that point, and until about thirty weeks, it seems that a decision concerning mourning could be made by the rabbi and the parents. There the actual length of the infant's life might become more of a factor than gestational age. In any event, burial is required, and that could serve as a focus of Jewish ritual.

At the moment, this issue of "how premature" remains unresolved. In its discussion, the CJLS apparently approved the opinion that any infant born alive no matter how premature, who remains alive for even the shortest amount of time, is treated as a full human being. In a dissenting concurrence, Rabbi Avram Reisner argues that following my primary halakhic reasoning of doubtful viability, we should retain the requirement of a certain gestational age (thirty weeks) before implementing full mourning practices as described in this rabbinic ruling. A premature infant born prior to that time, who dies before the end of thirty days, would continue to be treated as a miscarried fetus. . . .

Conclusion

It is an official position of the CJLS that in the case of neo-natal death—the death of a full-term or premature infant, prior to the completion of the thirtieth day of life—the death is treated in the same manner as we treat the death of someone who lived more than thirty days. That is: the body is treated and prepared as any Jewish body, there is burial and a funeral service (with readings and comments that are sensitive to the situation). The parents, and non-minor siblings, have the obligations of rending their clothes [as a sign of mourning], the period of *aninut* [between the death and the burial, with the special obligations of preparing for the burial], full mourning practices, including the seven-day mourning period of full mourning, reciting *kaddish* for thirty days, and observing *yahrzeit* [lighting a candle and saying *kaddish* on the anniversary of the death]. The community has all of its obligations for comforting mourners, including preparing the meal upon returning from the cemetery and providing a *minyan* [prayer quorum of ten Jewish adults] for *shivah* and beyond.[56]

As indicated by Rabbi Dickstein, Rabbi Avram Reisner dissented over the flexibility that she wanted to give local rabbis to decide when to require full mourning rites and when not to. He indicated his reasoning in a written dissent to Rabbi Dickstein's ruling:

I strongly support Rabbi Dickstein's view, proposed before her by Rabbi [Amy] Eilberg, that viability by today's medical standards should affect our understanding of the Amoraic [Talmudic Rabbis'] claim, "It is a virtual certainty that its gestation was complete." I challenged in committee, however, the flexible standard. I do not believe halakhah abides flexible standards. . . . I asked Rabbi Dickstein for a date certain. She was unwilling . . . to offer such. To wit, a child, born alive, even much smaller and younger than any reasonable viability standard, is the proper subject of mourning rites by this decision. . . .

. . . The measure that our sources attest is one of virtual certainty [that the child will live]. I propose that that measure is attained in our day at 31–32 weeks, that is, the end of the seventh month of gestation, when survival rates are greater than eighty-five percent according to Rabbi Dickstein's source (1986!), and certainly eighty percent according to the New York State Task Force report. At that point, it seems possible to say that it is a viable child with conviction. . . .

Let the completion of seven months, rather than the former nine, serve as the grounds for the claim of virtual certainty. Before that level of development let the old law stand that the child needs to prove viability by living thirty days to be considered a full legal person. That is what I believe we should rule.[57]

The issue motivating both Rabbis Dickstein and Reisner is the expectation of the parents that after the fifth month they will take home a baby that will live a normal life, even if he or she will need medical assistance during the first few weeks or months of life. It is the dashing of these presumptions, together with the dreams and hopes for the child that the parents by then already had, that needs to be mourned with the full support of traditional Jewish rites amid the comforting community. The dispute between Rabbis Dickstein and Reisner is only the time during the gestational period when the parents are likely to assume they will take home a healthy baby, which is Rabbi Dickstein's primary concern, and when contemporary medicine justifies that expectation, which is Rabbi Reisner's primary criterion. In any case, it is clear that unlike past eras, when parents were not sure that they had a viable child until thirty days after it was born, today that presumption comes even before birth—hence the discussion of adjusting traditional Jewish mourning rites to account for both the new medical ability to sustain prematurely born infants and the parents' presumptions based on this development.

Practical Advice for Neonatologists and Other Caregivers

In working with Jewish neonates and their parents, physicians and other caregivers should bear the following points in mind:

1. Jews vary in their attachments to Judaism, from ultra-Orthodox to secular, so the degree to which the Jewish tradition will play a role in how they respond to the care of neonates, and who will be trusted to interpret the Jewish tradition on this matter, will vary immensely, depending on the particular family's mode of Jewish identity. It is not improper and definitely worthwhile, therefore, to ask the parents how they identify as Jews—Hasidic (including Chabad), Modern Orthodox, Conservative, Reconstructionist, Reform, Renewal, or secular—as a way of understanding the relevance of the Jewish tradition and the way it will be interpreted in the care of the neonate.
2. The Jewish tradition, and Jews almost by osmosis, trust medicine and its practitioners, and Jews are generally aggressive in trying to preserve and protect both the quantity and quality of life. Therefore, do not be surprised if Jews, faced with bad news, ask for a second or even a third opinion.
3. That said, the Jewish tradition recognizes that we are mortal and that there are limits to what even the most well-trained human beings can do in saving a life. If the neonate really cannot be saved, reach out to the family's rabbi, if they have one, or a rabbi on the hospital staff to help the family cope with the need to accept the fact of the child's demise and to begin the mourning process.
4. As described earlier, rabbinic opinions vary, even within one movement (my example was the Conservative Movement)—not only on how aggressive medical personnel should be in trying to save even what will be a severely compromised life, but also on the proper mourning procedures for a neonate who dies. Here, the family's rabbi, if they have one, will be very

helpful in guiding the family in the proper burial rituals, in relieving any guilt they may have, warranted or not, and in organizing the family and community of mourners to help them cope with their loss.

Evolving Realities, Evolving Responses

As the science and technology regarding the treatment of neonates advance, we will increasingly have this question to answer: now that we can do x to keep a neonate alive, should we do that, even if it means that the person will live with major deficits? To some extent, this depends on medicine's advancing ability to sustain a child and to treat a child's medical and mental problems, and to some extent it is deeper than that, depending on how we evaluate quality of life and the degree to which that affects our judgment about extending its quantity. In addition to such moral dilemmas, religions will be called on to respond to the social and psychological issues involved—not only for the neonate but also for the parents and family. In all these ways, religions like Judaism will have to stretch to give moral guidance and psychological support in areas never traversed by our ancestors, at least to this degree. May we be wise enough to interpret and apply our varying religious traditions in the new ways that will make those traditions' vision of who we are and ought to be the powerful support that we look to them to be.

Notes

1. The following abbreviations for traditional Jewish sources are used:

> M. = Mishnah, edited c. 200 C.E.
> T. = Tosefta, edited c. 200 C.E.
> B. = Babylonian Talmud, edited c. 500 C.E.
> M.T. = Maimonides' *Mishneh Torah*, completed in 1177.
> S.A. = Joseph Karo's *Shulhan Arukh*, completed in 1663.

So, for example, state courts in Massachusetts (http://www.nytimes.com/1991/ 01/16/us/court-says-ill-child-s-interests-outweigh-religion.html, accessed February 14, 2014) and a number of other American states (http://jwdivorces.bravehost.com/ blood.html, accessed February 15, 2014), as well as the highest court in Canada (http://www.cbc.ca/news/canada/girl-s-forced-blood-transfusion-didn-t-violate-rights-top-court-1.858660, accessed February 14, 2014) and courts in Ireland (http:// www.religioustolerance.org/witness16.htm, accessed February 15, 2014), have ruled that parents must allow a blood transfusion for their child when medically necessary to keep the child alive despite the parents' (or even the teenage child's) religious objections based on their beliefs as Jehovah's Witnesses or Christian Scientists.

2. Immanuel Kant, *Religion within the Boundaries of Mere Reason*, 6:50, p. 94; Immanuel Kant, *Critique of Pure Reason* A548/B576, p. 473.

3. *Numbers Rabbah* 13:15–16. Throughout this essay, I will use the usual style in academic study of the Jewish tradition, referring to the classical rabbis of the Mishnah, Tosefta, Talmud, and Midrash as "the Rabbis," with an upper case R. They lived between the second century B.C.E. and the sixth century C.E., even though some of the books recording their opinions, especially in the texts of Midrash, were edited in later centuries. When referring to medieval and modern rabbis, I will use a lower case "r" (e.g., "rabbis in the Orthodox community"), unless I am using the word as the title of a particular person, followed by his or her proper name (e.g., Rabbi Joseph Karo).

4. Orthodox instructions for advance directives: http://www.rabbis.org/pdfs/hcpi.pdf. The Orthodox healthcare directive: http://www.rabbis.org/pdfs/FINAL_Revised_Halachic_Health_Care_Proxy.pdf. The Reform movement's approach to healthcare directives as appropriately the expression of an individual's will: http://www.urj.org/what-we-believe/resolutions/health-care-decisions-dying. Rabbi Richard Address, ed., *A Time to Prepare* (New York: Union of Reform Judaism, 1995, rtd. 2002); the advance directive in that book was written by Drs. Ezekiel and Linda Emanuel and was incorporated by Rabbi Address in his book as consistent with Reform ideology. The Conservative Movement's Advance Directive for Health Care: http://www.rabbinicalassembly.org/sites/default/files/public/halakhah/teshuvot/19861990/mackler_care.pdf (all accessed December 31, 2015).

5. Exodus 21:21–25. Catholic Bibles translate this differently because they are based on the Septuagint, a Greek translation of the Hebrew, which frankly misinterpreted the Hebrew.

6. M. *Bava Kamma* 8:1 and the Talmud thereon.

7. M. *Ohalot* 7:6.

8. T. *Shabbat* 16:4; B. *Shabbat* 135a; S.A. *Orah Hayyim* 330:7, 8; S.A. *Yoreh De'ah* 266:11. See also the lengthy discussion in this regard by R. Yitzhak Yaakov Weiss, *Minhat Yitzhak* 4, no. 12.

9. Jane E. Brody, "Rethinking 'Term Pregnancy,'" *New York Times*, November 11, 2013, accessed December 31, 2015, http://well.blogs.nytimes.com/2013/11/11/importance-of-on-time-deliveries/?_php=true&_type=blogs&_r=0, based on a more refined definitional structure of the period between thirty-seven and forty-one weeks of pregnancy (counting from the first day of the woman's last period before becoming pregnant) to indicate the differing outcomes expected in deliveries of babies in that period: "Definition of Term Pregnancy," The American College of Obstetrics and Gynecology, November 2013, accessed December 31, 2015, http://www.acog.org/About_ACOG/ACOG_Departments/~/media/Committee%20Opinions/Committee%20on%20Obstetric%20Practice/co579.pdf.

10. See the exception of Rabbi Avram Reisner's rabbinic ruling at note 29.

11. For a more extensive treatment of the fundamental convictions that underlie Judaism's approach to medicine generally, see Elliot N. Dorff, *Matters of Life and Death: A Jewish Approach to Modern Medical Ethics* (Philadelphia: Jewish Publication Society, 1998), Chapter Two.

12. That God causes illness as punishment for sin: Leviticus 26:14–16; Deuteronomy 28:22, 27, 58–61. That God heals us: Exodus 15:26; Deuteronomy 32:39; Isaiah 19:22; 57:18–19; Jeremiah 30:17; 33:6; Hosea 6:1; Psalms 103:2–3; 107:20: Job 5:18, etc.

13. Exodus 21:19; B. *Bava Kamma* 85a.

14. Deuteronomy 22:1–3; B. *Bava Kamma* 81b.

15. B. *Sanhedrin* 73a (using Leviticus 19:16), 84b (using Leviticus 19:18, and see Rashi's comment there).

16. Genesis 1:27; see also 5:1 and 9:6.

17. For a discussion on Jewish perceptions of and responses to disability, see Carl Astor, ". . . *Who Makes People Different*": *Jewish Perspectives on the Disabled* (New York: United Synagogue of America, 1985).

18. Genesis 3.

19. Ecclesiastes 3:2.

20. S.A. *Yoreh De'ah* 339:1.

21. J. David Bleich, *Judaism and Healing: Halakhic Perspectives* (New York: KTAV, 1981), Chapter 24. The citation is on p. 135.

22. http://www.rabbis.org/news/article.cfm?id=101022, accessed December 31, 2015. Rabbi Moshe Tendler wrote this position statement.

23. Fred Rosner, *Modern Medicine and Jewish Ethics* (Hoboken, NJ: KTAV and New York: Yeshiva University Press, 2nd revised edition, 1991), 209. I heard Rabbi Immanuel Jakobovits, the author of the first book on Jewish medical ethics and former Chief Rabbi of the United Kingdom, suggest this to a group of physicians at Cedars-Sinai Medical Center in Los Angeles in 1983.

24. http://www.rabbis.org/news/article.cfm?id=105607, accessed December 31, 2015.

25. Avram Israel Reisner, "A Halakhic Ethic for the Care of the Terminally Ill," *Conservative Judaism* 43, no. 3 (Spring 1991): 52–89; also at http://www. rabbinicalassembly.org/sites/default/files/public/halakhah/teshuvot/19861990/ reisner_care.pdf, accessed January 4, 2016.

26. Elliot N. Dorff, "A Jewish Approach to End-Stage Medical Care," *Conservative Judaism* 43, no. 3 (Spring 1991): 3–51; also at http://www.rabbinicalassembly.org/ sites/default/files/public/halakhah/teshuvot/19861990/dorff_care.pdf, accessed January 4, 2016.

27. Mark Washofsky, *Jewish Living: A Guide to Contemporary Reform Practice* (New York: UAHC, 2000), 250–51.

28. For a more developed account of these reasons to object to assisted suicide, see Dorff, *Matters of Life and Death* (at note 11 above), 176–98.

29. Avram Israel Reisner, "Peri- and Ne-Natology: The Matter of Limiting Treatment," p. 356, accessed January 4, 2016, http://www.rabbinicalassembly.org/sites/default/ files/public/halakhah/teshuvot/19912000/reisner_natology.pdf.

30. David A. Teutsch, *A Guide to Jewish Practice: Volume 1: Everyday Living* (Wyncote, PA: Reconstructionist Rabbinical College Press, 2011), 489.

31. Avraham Steinberg, M.D., *Encyclopedia of Jewish Medical Ethics,* trans. Fred Rosner, M.D. (Jerusalem and New York: Feldheim, 2003), 2:744.

32. See, for example, Washofsky, *Jewish Living* (at note 27 above), 250, for the Reform movement; and see Dorff, *Matters of Life and Death* (at note 11 above), 26–29,

184–86, 191–93, 201–02, 218–19 for a Conservative view of pain and the duty to alleviate it.

33. *Republic,* 5:460.

34. *Politics* 7, 16, 1334b–1336a.

35. Steinberg, *Encyclopedia of Jewish Medical Ethics* (at note 31 above), 747.

36. I know of several Jewish families who have adopted Chinese girls, and some years ago, the *New York Times* ran an article about the Bat Mitzvah of such a girl on its front page, "A Chinese Orphan's Journey to a Jewish Rite of Passage," March 8, 2007, A-1.

37. M. *Ketubbot* 4:9.

38. Exodus 21:18–19; M. *Bava Kamma* 8:1; B. *Bava Kamma* 85a.

39. For a discussion of how these two cases of distributing scarce resources can be applied in our day to determining who gets particular forms of health care and who pays for it, see Dorff, *Matters of Life and Death* (see note 11 above), Chapter Twelve.

40. See, for example, B. *Sanhedrin* 17b, where there is a list of the services that a city must have to enable a rabbinic scholar to live there.

41. Filial duties: B. *Kiddushin* 31b. Parental duties: B. *Kiddushin* 29a. For a discussion of both sets of duties, see Elliot N. Dorff, *Love Your Neighbor and Yourself: A Jewish Approach to Modern Personal Ethics* (Philadelphia: Jewish Publication Society, 2003), Chapter Four ("Parents and Children").

42. B. *Sotah* 14a.

43. B. *Nedarim* 39b–40a.

44. M.T. Laws of Mourning 14:4; see also S.A. *Yoreh De'ah* 335.

45. Elliot N. Dorff, *The Way into Tikkun Olam (Repairing the World)* (Woodstock, VT: Jewish Lights, 2005), 157–62.

46. B. *Pesaḥim* 64b; B. *Kiddushin* 39b.

47. B. *Avodah Zarah* 54b.

48. I would like to thank Professor Ronald M. Green for alerting me to this aspect of visiting parents.

49. Dorff, *The Way into Tikkun Olam (Repairing the World),* at note 45 above, 162–65.

50. S.A. *Yoreh De'ah* 340:30.

51. M. *Niddah* 5:3.

52. B. *Niddah* 44b.

53. S.A. *Yoreh De'ah* 344:4; Tractate Mourning, 186.

54. B. *Berakhot* 49a.

55. Rabbi Isodoro Aizenberg, "Mourning for a Newborn," accessed February 4, 2014, http://www.rabbinicalassembly.org/sites/default/files/public/halakhah/teshuvot/19861990/aizenberg_missingpersons.pdf.

56. Rabbi Stephanie Dickstein, "Jewish Ritual Practice following the Death of an Infant Who Lives Less than Thirty-One Days," accessed February 4, 2014, http://www.rabbinicalassembly.org/sites/default/files/public/halakhah/teshuvot/19912000/dickstein_infant.pdf.

57. Rabbi Avram Israel Reisner, "Kim Li: A Dissenting Concurrence," accessed February 4, 2014, http://www.rabbinicalassembly.org/sites/default/files/public/halakhah/teshuvot/19912000/reisner_kiyyamli.pdf.

2

Catholicism and the Neonatal Context

M. Therese Lysaught

On October 16, 2000, thirty-two weeks pregnant with twins, I sat in my office, preparing my lecture for the afternoon session of my undergraduate course entitled "Christian Ethics and Health Care." I had taught this course every semester for six years. I was preparing my remarks on a chapter I had taught almost every semester, the first chapter of Margaret Morhmann's short book, *Medicine as Ministry*.[1] Morhmann is a pediatric intensivist as well as a theologian-bioethicist who spent decades on faculty at the University of Virginia medical school, including an appointment in the Center for Biomedical Ethics and Humanities.

The first chapter of *Medicine as Ministry* is entitled "God Is One: The Temptations of Idolatry." Here, Morhmann explores the relationship between a central claim of the monotheistic faiths—that God is One—and our choices, decisions, and actions in the clinical context. She lifts up the Shema of the Jewish tradition—"Hear O Israel, the Lord our God, the Lord is One!"—and the first commandment of the Judeo-Christian tradition: "I am the Lord your God who brought you out of the land of Egypt, out of the house of slavery; You shall have no other gods before me."[2] She explores whether the current structures of medicine honor these claims, or whether they instead embody a deep idolatry—a worship of the false gods of medical technology or health or life or, perhaps, of the demiurge, death.[3] In support of her challenge, she quotes Mother Teresa, elaborating on an observation the saint once made upon visiting a neonatal intensive care unit (NICU) in the United States:

> Mother Teresa, for one, has called the neonatal intensive care units that populate American hospitals "obscene"; she could as easily have called them "blasphemous."[4]

I took great pleasure in teaching this passage because undergraduates of all stripes generally love Mother Teresa. Consequently, they are quite taken aback to hear her criticize something that seems, on its face, to be so good—neonatal medicine. That afternoon, I was ready yet again to hit them with this challenge, to shake up their given conceptual frameworks, and to demonstrate how theology can destabilize taken-for-granted assumptions and open up new as-yet-unasked questions.

I never made it to class. Twenty-four hours later, I found myself sitting between two isolettes in the NICU of Kettering Medical Center—a hospital in the Seventh-day Adventist tradition—isolettes that housed my two newly born, two-month-premature babies. Like most parents of preemies, I had never expected my babies to arrive early. I had never expected to be whisked into the high-tech world of neonatal medicine, to sit on the sidelines while others monitored and managed a dizzying array of my children's bodily functions and overall well-being, to be consulted on a daily basis as the de jure decision maker, rubber-stamping in my hormone-bathed mental state the daily recommendations of the truly outstanding neonatal care team.

But, unlike most parents of preemies, I sat amid this whirlwind not only as a mother but also as a Catholic moral theologian and medical ethicist. I had taught cases akin to many that populated the other isolettes around me. I knew well the principles that applied—both the principles of biomedical ethics and the principles of the Catholic moral tradition. And as I sat there day after day for almost a month, I found myself saying a number of times: "Mother Teresa says this is obscene. Margaret Mohrmann suggests it might be blasphemous."

Needless to say, it was a rather surreal experience to be a Catholic theologian, a medical ethicist, *and* the mother of premature twins all in the same moment. It was akin to being both a vulnerable refugee in a strange country where one neither speaks the language nor knows the customs and being an anthropologist among the natives or an embedded journalist, all at the same time. My brain oscillated between the biologically driven compulsion to do everything so that my children would survive—all the while analyzing, observing, documenting, critiquing.

After the children came home, the anthropologist was put on the backburner. There were more pressing things to deal with than the practical, theological, and ethical dynamics of the NICU. My reflections in this chapter mark the first time I have written about neonatal medicine since that unexpected immersion experience. In what follows, I leave most of my anthropological insights to the side. Yet, my NICU experience as a mother-theologian-scholar inevitably lies in the background whenever I approach these questions. And, while sharing many commonalities, this experience was not like that of all NICU parents: apart from being born at thirty-two weeks, my children were never really in any grave peril, at least as far as we knew. True, my son was not breathing and may not have had a heartbeat when he was born, but the excellent staff remedied that rather quickly. My daughter had a pneumothorax, but it resolved itself within 24 hours. The children were small but not tiny—1,640 and 1,950 grams, respectively—chubby babies by NICU standards. They mostly needed to learn how to eat and fatten up so that they could self-regulate their body temperatures. My daughter eventually needed an apnea monitor, but truth be told, it made those first months of parenting easier. They stayed at the hospital for roughly three weeks. And they have no developmental or other sorts of disabilities. They are healthy, athletic, smart, and flourishing. Thus, our experience was neither one of critical ethical dilemmas nor negative sequelae.

Catholicism and Neonatal Medicine: Contours and Complexities

In this chapter, I have been asked to focus on one very specific topic: Catholicism in the neonatal context. As the editors of this volume have noted, currently, there is little or no literature available within the discipline of biomedical ethics to assist neonatal caregivers in understanding how religious beliefs and values might influence parents' responses to the challenges posed by their newborn's care.[5] Equally, there is little or no literature available within the disciplines of academic or pastoral theology addressing questions of neonatal medicine. My contribution here seeks to address the question: in what ways might the teachings and religious practices of the Roman Catholic tradition inform the ways in which parents and caregivers make treatment decisions about the high-risk newborn infant?

Let me begin by providing some background on Catholicism in the United States. For decades, Catholics have comprised approximately 22% of the US population, with approximately seventy million Catholics living in the United States today.[6] This makes Roman Catholicism the largest single religious denomination in the United States. Although Catholic presence varies geographically, a sizeable proportion of the patient census in most hospitals will likely be Catholic. The growing edge of the Roman Catholic Church in the United States is the Hispanic or Latino Catholic population; as of February 2013, nearly half of Catholics in the United States younger than forty years were Hispanic (46%). This cohort is of childbearing age. Given ongoing issues of access to health care (even with the Affordable Care Act), compounded by immigration politics and the socioeconomics of race, many women in this cohort will continue to receive inadequate prenatal care, resulting in potentially higher rates of prematurity and other issues that will land them and their babies in the NICU.

Thus, a significant number of Catholics make their way through the doors of the NICU in the United States. On simply a percentage basis, roughly 125,000 premature babies born each year in the United States will have a Catholic parent. Yet, simply because a patient or family identifies with a particular religious tradition does not mean that the teachings, beliefs, and practices of that tradition necessarily influence their actions and decisions or influence the actions and decisions of all members of a tradition in the same way. There is a preponderance of Catholics in the United States, but the ways in which these seventy million people inhabit Catholicism certainly vary.

Immigrants and foreign visitors aside, American Catholics—just like most of the rest of the people who walk into the clinical setting—are often more deeply formed and informed by the traditions of US culture, their profession, and their socioeconomic class than by their faith tradition. For example, while civil divorce is generally considered a grave, morally illicit offense per Catholic teaching,[7] divorce rates among Catholics are lower than other groups in the United States, but not by an overwhelming margin.[8] Catholics cite lower rates of abortion than their Protestant counterparts in the United States, reflecting the Catholic Church's opposition to abortion, but again not by a large margin.[9] Pew Research in 2013 found that roughly 50% of Catholics support both same-sex marriage and keeping abortion legal.[10]

Like many long-lived religious traditions, one finds a spectrum of adherence. Roughly 40% of Catholics attend Mass on a weekly basis; 17% go "seldom or never," with the remaining 43% all over the map.[11] Various groups adhere strongly to one part of the tradition or another. There are the visibly evangelical Catholics who identify with the Church's teachings on marriage and life so much so that we used to be able to say they were "right of the Pope." There are the social justice Catholics who are passionate about the Church's social justice tradition but have no time or patience for the Church's teachings on marriage and sexuality. There is a sizeable middle ground who are deeply faithful in practice and who do their best to hold both of these poles together. There are those who pray the rosary and believe in Marian apparitions; there are those who join the Maryknolls and do mission work in Central and South America. Then add the immigrant populations, where Catholic belief and practice have been interwoven for centuries with particular cultural traditions, and it gets very complex. Or, as we often say, Catholicism is a Big Tent.

Yet, Catholicism does present one decided advantage over many other religious traditions: Catholicism has developed an authoritative body of literature on key questions related to medicine and health care to which clinicians, the faithful, and others can turn for (relatively) clear guidance. In addition to a two-thousand-year tradition of saints, theologians, and developing wisdom, Catholics have a century's worth of papal encyclicals, apostolic exhortations, pastoral letters, and other documents issued by authoritative persons or bodies to which we can refer to try to clarify what the Church actually teaches on a given topic.

For the purposes of this chapter, I will draw largely from one very short document, *The Ethical and Religious Directives for Catholic Health Care Services.*[12] The *ERDs*, as they are often called, distill in pamphlet form basic convictions of the Catholic tradition and a set of directives or guidelines that provide the parameters for the ethical practice of medicine within Catholic healthcare institutions. The *ERDs* are designed to be a resource for all who work in Catholic health care as well as for patients and families who wish to make decisions consistent with their Catholic faith while situated in other-than-Catholic healthcare contexts.

Additionally, over the past two millennia, Catholicism has developed a rich and extensive set of liturgical traditions that are deeply inhabited by most Catholics. Sacramental practices, augmented by artifacts of material culture (such as images of Our Lady of Guadalupe for Latino/a Catholics or the Sacred Heart of Jesus for Catholics of European descent), are critical resources for many Catholics in times of illness, discernment, and death. When faced with a medical crisis, even Catholics who seldom attend Mass—or who may not have set foot in a church for decades—will instinctively turn to the sacraments and rites of the Church for comfort, for strength, for tradition, or for reasons unknown even to them.

Thus, demographically, "Catholicism" is not a monolithic entity but, rather, provides a complex and varied landscape; theologically and liturgically, Catholicism is a richly contoured tradition that provides a multiplicity of resources for patients, families, and caregivers to draw on. In the NICU, this complex and contoured religious tradition meets an equally multifaceted clinical reality. Neonatal cases vary widely. Charles Camosy, in his book, *Too Expensive to Treat? Finitude, Tragedy, and the Neonatal ICU*, helpfully groups neonatal patients into four categories:

- Full-term babies with acute illnesses
- Babies with congenital anomalies
- Babies with prematurity
- Babies with extreme prematurity

The types of issues encountered with neonatal patients may vary from category to category. While it would be most useful to examine how the Roman Catholic tradition might be applied to specific cases in the previous categories, in what follows, I will primarily provide an overview of the teachings and practices of the Roman Catholic tradition that are broadly applicable across categories. Ideally, readers of this volume could meet together with their pastoral care and ethics staff to explore how these teachings and practices might illuminate specific cases they have encountered in their own clinical contexts.

Roman Catholic Principles in the Neonatal Setting

For caregivers working with Catholic parents and decision makers in the neo-natal setting, seven fundamental convictions or areas of teaching of the Roman Catholic tradition would be most relevant: (1) understandings of the moral and religious status of the premature infant or newborn; (2) teaching on patient deci-sion making; (3) guidelines regarding withholding and withdrawing treatment; (4) developments with regard to medically assisted nutrition and hydration; (5) teaching on the care and treatment of conditions considered incompatible with life; (6) advocacy of palliative care; and (7) teaching on the care of dead bodies, including burial, autopsy, and organ donation.

The Dignity of the Human Person

Despite the variety of ways Catholics inhabit their tradition, it is safe to say that most Catholics are grasped by a deep, almost embodied commitment to the value of human life and the dignity of the human person.[13] This conviction will be an operative factor in the discernment process of many Catholic parents. Especially with the papacy of John Paul II, this unwavering commitment to the dignity of the human person and the sanctity of human life gained a new visibility. For the *ERDs*, it is the foundational principle.

First, Catholic healthcare ministry is rooted in a commitment to promote and defend human dignity; this is the foundation of its concern to respect the sacred-ness of every human life from the moment of conception until death. The first right of the human person, the right to life, entails a right to the means for the proper development of life, such as adequate health care.[14]

Within Catholicism, there is a spectrum of adherence to this conviction. At one end are the vitalists, who insist on maintaining human biological life under any and all conditions, at any and all costs (a position not exclusive to Catholicism, by the way). As we will see later, the Catholic tradition is *not* vitalist, but there are self-identified Catholics who inhabit this position. At the other end of the spectrum are those, such as Catholics for Choice (formerly known as Catholics for Free Choice), who engage in advocacy efforts to advance access to safe and legal abortion services.[15]

Most Catholics inhabit a middle ground—they see human life as a holy thing, a unique image of God, and see each living person as having inherent dignity and worth regardless of social location, disability, age, health status, and so on. Importantly, the Catholic tradition does *not* define "personhood" as consisting in certain capacities or even potential for capacities, as is often the case in secular bioethics. From the moment of conception until "natural death," each and every human being *is* considered to be a *person*, a creature of God, someone loved by God and therefore to be loved by us, regardless of their social utility, the costs of their care, how "disabled" they might be, or what potential for such disability there might be.[16] In fact, there is a sense in the Catholic tradition that the more vulnerable a person is, the greater the obligation to treat them with respect and dignity.

Most parents—Catholic or not—understand their neonate to be not only a *baby* but also a *person*.[17] This perspective will shape the ways in which they care for their infant as well as the decisions they make about treatment options. They will generally expect hospital staff to do the same, regardless of their baby's condition. It is encouraging to see the evolution of language used with regard to neonatal patients, at least within the field of bioethics. No longer discussed under the heading of "handicapped newborns" or "defective neonates," the language has shifted to "the high-risk neonatal patient." This change in language signals a conceptual advance that sees the child not primarily as *defective* but, rather, hopefully, as a patient with inherent dignity and worth. In all interactions with neonatal patients and their families, the Catholic tradition would encourage all caregivers to envisage and treat neonates as unique persons of value and to support parents as they do the same.

Patient Decision Making in Catholic Perspective

How do or ought religious beliefs factor into patient decision making from a Catholic perspective? Some, at times, wish to draw a dichotomy between "autonomy" and "heteronomy" in moral decision making. A Catholic perspective would challenge drawing this distinction too sharply. Contra Kant, all morality really is heteronomous. It is a rare (or perhaps nonexistent) moral principle or moral framework that a person can make up oneself. With few exceptions, we all adopt moral principles from "outside" ourselves. Consider the principle of utility, for example—John Stuart Mill coined this one, and most of us have imbibed it as an eternal truth from our culture. It often possesses a power over us that is difficult to resist. So it is with all moral principles. Especially because morality inherently has a social function, all morality is heteronomous. Thus, patient decision making across traditions is much more nuanced than either heteronomy or autonomy—and therefore more complicated and messy.

The *ERDs* understand the patient–physician relationship—and therefore the decision-making process—to be a collaborative endeavor. The Bishops open Part Three of the *ERDs*, entitled "The Professional-Patient Relationship," with a rich account of this mutual collaboration:

A person in need of health care and the professional health care provider who accepts that person as a patient enter into a relationship that requires, among other things, mutual respect, trust, honesty, and appropriate confidentiality. The resulting free exchange of information must avoid manipulation, intimidation, or condescension. Such a relationship enables the patient to disclose personal information needed for effective care and permits the health care provider to use his or her professional competence most effectively to maintain or restore the patient's health. Neither the health care professional nor the patient acts independently of the other; both participate in the healing process.[18]

It is within this shared context that the Catholic tradition locates the centrality of voluntary, informed patient decision-making. As the *ERDs* note:

Free and informed consent requires that the person or the person's surrogate receive all reasonable information about the essential nature of the proposed treatment and its benefits; its risks, side-effects, consequences, and cost; and any reasonable and morally legitimate alternatives, including no treatment at all.

Each person or the person's surrogate should have access to medical and moral information and counseling so as to be able to form his or her conscience.[19]

What we hear here is that patients—or, in the neonatal context, patients' families—are charged with the task of making *informed* decisions. These decisions should be informed by a variety of sources. The medical facts and economic realities are first and foremost. In deciding whether to pursue a particular treatment, parents are enjoined to take into consideration "its benefits; its risks, side-effects, consequences, and cost." Health care professionals are enjoined to provide this information to parents in a way they can understand and in a nonbiased manner.

This empirical information enters into the ongoing process of formation of conscience. Conscience is considered almost sacrosanct within the Catholic tradition. It is that central human intellectual and moral faculty that interprets and reasons through particular situations in light of moral principles. In the words of the Second Vatican Council, "Conscience is the most secret core and sanctuary of a man. There he is alone with God, Whose voice echoes in his depths."[20] One's conscience must be formed well in order to function well. Ideally, conscience is formed on an ongoing basis by information, prayer, and consultation with others—family, friends, healthcare professionals, and clergy. Relevant information includes medical and economic information as well as familial and social commitments and Church teachings.

Thus, religious beliefs should enter into parental decision making in the neonatal context as one component of a careful process of reasoned discernment, or perhaps as an integrative framework that helps structure how the various components are related to each other. Such a decision-making process is far from formulaic. While communal and collaborative, the ultimate decision is finally the province of the patient or, in this case, the patient's parents. In this way, the Catholic respect for the dignity of the human person translates into a respect for conscience, productively integrating what might otherwise be construed as autonomy and heteronomy.[21]

Withholding and Withdrawing Treatment

Most Catholics are quite familiar with the Church's teaching on the dignity of the human person and conscience. Many, however, are not aware of the Church's teaching on withholding and withdrawing treatment; many others misunderstand it. Against those who take a vitalist position, Directive 28 makes clear that a viable treatment option may be "no treatment at all."

The Catholic tradition on withholding and withdrawing treatment is a clear, nuanced, well-established, five-hundred-year old position. It is summed up succinctly in the *ERDs*:

> A person has a moral obligation to use ordinary or proportionate means of preserving his or her life. Proportionate means are those that in the judgment of the patient offer a reasonable hope of benefit and do not entail an excessive burden or impose excessive expense on the family or the community.
>
> A person may forgo extraordinary or disproportionate means of preserving life. Disproportionate means are those that in the patient's judgment do not offer a reasonable hope of benefit or entail an excessive burden, or impose excessive expense on the family or the community.[22]

These two Directives succinctly capture key convictions:

- Human life is a fundamental good—a gift, a holy thing! If it can be saved or prolonged using *reasonable* means, one has a moral obligation to do so.
- The locus of decision making is, again, the patient, or in the neonatal context, the parents.
- "Benefit," notably, is not defined; it is not limited to a "reasonable hope of extending biological life." What constitutes "benefit" is left to the judgment of the patient; the assessment of benefit must be *reasonable*, but the

Directives make clear that benefit is determined relative to the medical condition and conscience of the patient.

- Likewise, "burden" is not defined. It must simply not be *excessive*, and
  reasons should be given for that judgment.
- Expense to the patient's family or community may legitimately be taken
  into account, even rendering an "ordinary" means "extraordinary."
- Human persons are finite; death is an inevitable reality for all.
- And last, medical treatments may be declined or removed. Not all "means
  of preserving life" are morally obligatory.

Within this framework, those interventions that offer a reasonable hope of benefit *and* reasonable burden and cost are *always* obligatory. One should always
pursue the good if one can, within reason. But note the conjunctions in the directives. One has no obligation to pursue treatments if one of the conditions does
not obtain: if there is not a reasonable hope of benefit; *or* if the burdens would be
excessive; *or* if the intervention would impose excessive expense on the family or
community.

Benefit and burden have long been understood broadly in the Catholic tradition. A patient is permitted to take into account psychological, social, spiritual,
familial, and financial dimensions of any treatment protocol. Pope Pius XII clarified two additional nuances in 1957, noting:

> But normally one is held to use only ordinary means—according to
> circumstances of persons, places, times, and culture—that is to say, means that
> do not involve any grave burden for oneself or another. A more strict obligation
> would be too burdensome for most men and would render the attainment of
> the higher, more important goods too difficult. Life, health, all temporal activi-
> ties are in fact subordinated to spiritual ends. On the other hand, one is not for-
> bidden to take more than the strictly necessary steps to preserve life and health,
> as long as he does not fail in some more serious duty. . . . On the other hand,
> since these forms of treatment go beyond the ordinary means to which one is
> bound, it cannot be held that there is an obligation to use them nor, conse-
> quently, that one is bound to give the doctor permission to use them.[23]

Per the Pontiff, a *medical means* is not ordinary or extraordinary in and of itself;
that determination is based in part on the patient's overall circumstances. And,
in keeping with the Thomistic tradition of Catholicism, Pius identifies a hierarchy of goods, with the physical goods of health and even life being subordinated to—and "ordered to"—the pursuit of spiritual ends.

Human life is a great and wonderful good—sacred, sanctified, with inherent
dignity. It is to be loved, respected, protected, and promoted. But it is *not an*

absolute.[24] As natural death draws near, it is not obligatory to prolong biological life at all (or even significant) costs. As the Vatican noted in its 1980 *Declaration on Euthanasia*, refusal of disproportionate treatment "is not the equivalent of suicide" but rather "should be considered an acceptance of the human condition."[25] This document affirms that patients may withhold or withdraw certain forms of medical treatment that "would only secure a precarious and burdensome prolongation of life." The *Catechism of the Catholic Church* suggests that to fight death "at all costs" may in fact be morally problematic:

> Discontinuing medical procedures that are burdensome, dangerous, extraordinary, or disproportionate to the expected outcome can be legitimate; it is the refusal of "over-zealous" treatment. Here one does not will to cause death; one's inability to impede it is merely accepted. The decisions should be made by the patient if he is competent and able or, if not, by those legally entitled to act for the patient, whose reasonable will and legitimate interests must always be respected.[26]

The *Catechism* here highlights one of the points of tension within the application of Catholic teaching on withholding and withdrawing treatment. For the teaching, as it developed over most of its five-hundred-year history, presumed the patient would be the one making the calculation about burdens and benefits relative to herself or himself. For most of this five-hundred-year history, there were few decisions to be made by families about patients. Over the past forty years—and particularly in the neonatal setting—this has changed dramatically. And this is where it becomes the most difficult. It is one thing for a patient to decline a course of treatment because it may impose excessive expense on his family; how can a surrogate make that same decision without devaluing the life of the neonate because he or she is disabled or expensive or inconvenient?

Thus, in practice, in the neonatal setting, definitions of benefit and burden have necessarily narrowed somewhat. In all instances, the Catholic tradition holds, "those whose lives are diminished or weakened deserve special respect. Sick or handicapped persons should be helped to lead lives as normal as possible."[27] Thus, if a medical intervention can help move a child toward a reasonable level of functioning—even with disability, expense, and ongoing medical support—that intervention may well be ordinary and obligatory. If a medical intervention promises little benefit in terms of advancing function *or* would impose an excessive burden *on the patient* or is proving *excessively* expensive to the family, then it may well be extraordinary and not required.

Such evaluations must be made by parents in collaborative consultation with the medical staff, family, friends, and perhaps even clergy based on the good of the patient and the patient's best interests. But the good of the child and the good of the parents are deeply intertwined. We see this acknowledged, again, by Pius XII in his address cited earlier, where he comments on the morality of discontinuing resuscitation:

> The rights and duties of the family [with regard to decision-making] depend in general upon the presumed will of the unconscious patient if he is of age and *sui juris*. Where the proper and independent duty of the family is concerned, they are usually bound only to the use of ordinary means . . . . Consequently, if it appears that the attempt at resuscitation constitutes in reality such a burden for the family that one cannot in all conscience impose it upon them, they can lawfully insist that the doctor should discontinue these attempts, and the doctor can lawfully comply. There is not involved here a case of direct disposal of the life of the patient, nor of euthanasia in any way: this would never be licit. Even when it causes the arrest of circulation, the interruption of attempts at resuscitation is never more than an indirect cause of the cessation of life, and one must apply in this case the principle of double effect and of "voluntarium in causa."

While Catholic teaching on withholding and withdrawing treatment does not mandate extraordinary treatment, it also does not prohibit it. Parents may validly choose for their children what others may consider to be extraordinary treatments. While futile or vitalist interventions are discouraged by the Catholic tradition, caring for the disabled may be understood as a powerful form of witness. Families who choose to care for children with significant health issues ought to be supported by the communities in which they are located.

Medically Assisted Nutrition and Hydration

Few are not aware of the battles that have raged within the Catholic tradition over the past fifteen years around the question of medically assisted nutrition and hydration (MANH). For the most part, the argument has focused on patients in persistent vegetative state.[28] How might Church teaching on MANH apply to the neonatal context?

Until 2009, Catholic teaching on MANH generally followed the overall guidelines for withholding and withdrawing treatment outlined previously. But, subsequent to the Terri Schiavo case, and a brief address by Pope John Paul II to a conference on "Life Sustaining Treatments and the Vegetative State" held at the Vatican in 2004, the issue of MANH has become more contested. In this address, John Paul II stated:

I should like particularly to underline how the administration of water and food, even when provided by artificial means, always represents a *natural means* of preserving life, not a *medical act*. Its use, furthermore, should be considered, in principle, *ordinary* and *proportionate*, and as such morally obligatory, insofar as and until it is seen to have attained its proper finality, which in the present case consists in providing nourishment to the patient and alleviation of his suffering.[29]

Some were concerned that in seeming to name a particular medical intervention as ordinary and proportionate in all situations, John Paul II was contradicting five hundred years of Catholic tradition. Yet, a more careful reading of the statement in context allays concerns. Importantly, the document applies only to patients in persistent vegetative states. To take this passage out of context and apply it to all patients would be a misinterpretation of the document.

At issue is the normal care due to the sick; Catholic teaching is clear that one must never abandon care for a seriously ill or dying patient. In many cases, the initiation of MANH in patients in crisis is the standard of practice; it is a standard intervention in the neonatal setting, usually intended as a short-term intervention designed to bridge neonates to the point at which they can develop the sucking reflex and coordinate sucking and swallowing (approximately thirty-four weeks' gestational age). For some impaired newborns, however, MANH becomes permanent. For severely impaired newborns, or those whose medical issues become critical before thirty-four weeks, questions may be raised about discontinuing tube feeding.

Directive 58 of the *ERDs* provides the parameters for addressing such situations. As the Bishops note:

In principle, there is an obligation to provide patients with food and water, including medically assisted nutrition and hydration for those who cannot take food orally. This obligation extends to patients in chronic and presumably irreversible conditions (e.g., the "persistent vegetative state") who can reasonably be expected to live indefinitely if given such care. Medically assisted nutrition and hydration become morally optional when they cannot reasonably be expected to prolong life or when they would be "excessively burdensome for the patient or [would] cause significant physical discomfort, for example resulting from complications in the use of the means employed." For instance, as a patient draws close to inevitable death from an underlying progressive and fatal condition, certain measures to provide nutrition and hydration may become excessively burdensome and therefore not obligatory in light of their very limited ability to prolong life or provide comfort.[30]

The Directive sets the question within the fundamental context, namely, that (in the words of the *Catechism*), "those whose lives are diminished or weakened deserve special respect. Sick or handicapped persons should be helped to lead lives as normal as possible."[31] In most situations, the administration of nutrition and hydration—either through traditional means or medically assisted—provides reasonable benefit with reasonable burden; in most situations it is *ordinary* and therefore obligatory. But circumstances can change. The same intervention that initially was ordinary may, because of the changing situation of the patient, become "morally optional" or extraordinary. If MANH—alone or in conjunction other interventions—becomes, in the estimation of the parents, excessively burdensome for the patient, or if the usual battery of medical interventions does little more than impede death, MANH may become morally optional.

Fundamentally, the main question is: what is the purpose or aim of the withdrawal of MANH or any other intervention? Is the treatment being removed because it is not effective or because it is imposing an excessive burden on the patient? Or is it being removed in order that the patient will die? At issue here is the intention and the real goal or end. The Catholic tradition retains a commitment to the distinction between allowing death to come versus deciding for death (a.k.a., euthanasia, assisted suicide). Euthanasia, as defined by the Catholic tradition, is "an action or an omission which of itself or *by intention causes* death, *in order that* all suffering may in this way be eliminated."[32] In other words, it is legitimate to withdraw treatment if there is a problem with the treatment (insufficient benefit, excessive burden); it is not legitimate to withdraw treatment because there is a problem with the patient (impairment or suffering). It is legitimate not to fight death at all costs; it is not legitimate to bring death forward.

At work here are two aspects of the Catholic tradition often obscured by our culture. The first is that the Catholic moral tradition is more one of *character* than of *consequences*. The Catholic moral tradition has for centuries forwarded a virtue ethic, an ethic that evaluates actions based not only on their outcomes or consequences on others or in the world but equally based on their effect on the character of the agent. Premised on a complex account of human moral psychology, all actions are understood to have a reciprocal effect on the person who commits them. All actions we commit are understood to shape us—our wills, our dispositions, our bodies, the interpretive lens through which we view the world—in particular directions, toward or away from certain fundamental goods. In doing so, each action trains us more easily to commit similar actions in the future. The more I commit a particular action, the more it becomes a habit.

This character or virtue framework informs Catholic teaching on end-of-life care. A key question is: how will a particular end-of-life action affect the character of the decision maker? Acts of euthanasia, where an agent actively pursues or brings forward death (an end that diminishes human flourishing), are understood to habituate that person to more easily carry out further acts of killing. They habituate and reinforce certain character traits—efficiency, expediency, control—that may be at odds with fundamental Christian virtues. Allowing a patient to die, when death is imminent, however, is understood to aim toward a different goal and inculcate a different set of virtues. To accept death's imminence is not to aim toward or to seek death; it is, rather, to simply acknowledge an inescapable part of reality. To allow death to come often requires actions that inculcate the virtues of patience (death often will not be hurried or work on our own timetable), of charity (the gift of self offered by being present to the patient through attention and caregiving), of hospitality (welcoming the patient despite his or her anomalies or impairments), or of prudence (as one constantly evaluates care options in the face of the patient's demise).

Thus, actions and decisions in the neonatal context ought (from a Catholic perspective) to be evaluated in part relative to the effects of those actions on the character of medical staff and parents. The Catholic tradition also challenges those in the neonatal context to evaluate the lens through which they perceive imperiled patients. It pushes back against what has often been perceived as a subtle but advancing cultural lens that values efficiency, economics, and control over the lives of human persons. This mindset is at times referred to as the "culture of death." Pope John Paul II in his 1995 encyclical *Evangelium Vitae* describes this mindset as:

> . . . a veritable structure of sin. This reality is characterized by the emergence of a culture which denies solidarity and in many cases takes the form of a veritable "culture of death." This culture is actively fostered by powerful cultural, economic and political currents which encourage an idea of society excessively concerned with efficiency. Looking at the situation from this point of view, it is possible to speak in a certain sense of a war of the powerful against the weak: a life which would require greater acceptance, love and care is considered useless, or held to be an intolerable burden, and is therefore rejected in one way or another. A person who, because of illness, handicap or, more simply, just by existing, compromises the well-being or life-style of those who are more favoured tends to be looked upon as an enemy to be resisted or eliminated. In this way a kind of "conspiracy against life" is unleashed.[33]

While it is true that the taking of life not yet born or in its final stages is sometimes marked by a mistaken sense of altruism and human compassion, it cannot be denied that such a culture of death, taken as a whole, betrays an individualistic concept of freedom, which ends up by becoming the freedom of "the strong" against the weak, who have no choice but to submit.[34]

For John Paul II, the culture of death is a subtle force, driven by powerful yet often invisible economic factors and masked by "a mistaken sense of compassion," which justifies eliminating persons with illness and disabilities. Persons with disability complicate society's drive toward ever-greater efficiency, productivity, and economic growth. Yet, within a Catholic perspective, *our* personhood—the personhood of the strong—calls us toward a greater solidarity with those who are vulnerable, poor, weak, and in need. As the *ERDs* note,

> Catholic health care should distinguish itself by service to and advocacy for those people whose social condition puts them at the margins of our society and makes them particularly vulnerable to discrimination. . . . In particular, the person with mental or physical disabilities, regardless of the cause or severity, must be treated as a unique person of incomparable worth, with the same right to life and to adequate health care as all other persons.[35]

Neonatal medicine is one of the first instances of this solidarity in the lives of most high-risk infants.

Persons or Conditions? Conditions "Incompatible with Life"

Catholic teaching and theologians have rarely addressed questions of infants with conditions deemed "incompatible with life," presuming that the principles outlined earlier are sufficient. However, questions surrounding the treatment of anencephalic fetuses have been disputed within the Catholic tradition for at least the past thirty years.[36] The main areas of disagreement have primarily concerned prenatal interventions—namely, is it morally licit to terminate a pregnancy once a diagnosis of anencephaly is made?

The US Catholic Bishops weighed in definitively on this question in 1996 with their statement, "Moral Principles Concerning Infants with Anencephaly."[37] Reaffirming the dignity and personhood of anencephalic fetuses, they concluded that:

> It is clear that before "viability" it is never permitted to terminate the gestation of an anencephalic child as the *means* of avoiding psychological or physical risks to the mother. Nor is such termination permitted after "viability" if early delivery endangers the child's life due to complications of prematurity. . . . Only if the complications of the pregnancy result in a life-threatening pathology of the mother, may the treatment of this pathology be permitted even at a risk to the child, and then only if the child's death is not a means to treating the mother.

Yet, the Bishops are not vitalists. They do not argue that, postpartum, all efforts to extend the biological life of anencephalic infants ought to be employed. Rather, they affirm the practice of solidarity as noted previously:

> The anencephalic child during his or her probably brief life after birth should be given the comfort and palliative care appropriate to all the dying. This failing life need not be further troubled by using extraordinary means to prolong it. It is most commendable for parents to wish to donate the organs of an anencephalic child for transplants that may assist other children, but this may never be permitted before the donor child is certainly dead.

This reasoning would apply to other infants with congenital conditions that are generally fatal within the first month of life, such as Meckel-Gruber syndrome, various chromosomal abnormalities, Potter syndrome, and Trisomies 13 and 18. For conditions such as Tay-Sachs disease, in which symptom onset is later, reasonable medical treatment would be indicated, following Directives 57 and 58.

Palliative Care

Catholic teaching on conditions "incompatible with life" signals the importance of palliative care in the neonatal context. Palliative care in the neonatal or perinatal setting remains a growing edge of this important movement within medicine. Ideally, palliative medicine should become a norm in the neonatal context, insofar as new developments in palliative medicine reject the former distinction between "doing everything" for the patient and "doing nothing but pain management" (hospice). Palliative medicine, as it is now understood, has expanded beyond only end-of-life care to the holistic treatment of all patients with life-threatening or chronic diseases.[38]

The World Health Organization (WHO) definition of palliative care captures its many dimensions.[39] Recently, the WHO has further articulated what palliative medicine means specifically in the care of children, noting:

> Palliative care for children represents a special, albeit closely related field to adult palliative care. WHO's definition of palliative care appropriate for children and their families is as follows; the principles apply to other paediatric chronic disorders:
>
> • Palliative care for children is the active total care of the child's body, mind and spirit, and also involves giving support to the family.

- It begins when illness is diagnosed, and continues regardless of whether or not a child receives treatment directed at the disease.
- Health providers must evaluate and alleviate a child's physical, psychological, and social distress.
- Effective palliative care requires a broad multidisciplinary approach that includes the family and makes use of available community resources; it can be successfully implemented even if resources are limited.
- It can be provided in tertiary care facilities, in community health centres and even in children's homes.[40]

Thus, consistent with the broader field, palliative care in the neonatal context should be provided to all neonatal patients; it does not signal that the patient is necessarily terminal and entails equally care for the patient's family.

Out of concerns about euthanasia and the culture of death, some within the Catholic tradition have been slow to accept the validity of palliative care in general.[41] Yet, many Catholic hospitals have been leading the way in implementing palliative care, given its deep resonance with the best of the Catholic tradition,[42] and Catholic magisterial writings have recently affirmed the importance of palliative care. As the *Catechism* notes:

> Even if death is thought imminent, the ordinary care owed to a sick person cannot be legitimately interrupted. The use of painkillers to alleviate the sufferings of the dying, even at the risk of shortening their days, can be morally in conformity with human dignity if death is not willed as either an end or a means, but only foreseen and tolerated as inevitable. Palliative care is a special form of disinterested charity. As such it should be encouraged.[43]

Similarly, the work of Pope-Emeritus Benedict XVI highlights the convergence between the WHO definition of palliative care and the Catholic tradition. Benedict names palliative care as "a right belonging to every human being, one which we must all be committed to defend."[44] He sees it as providing "integral care, offering the sick the human assistance and spiritual accompaniment they need."[45] And he understands palliative care as a medical practice inextricably tied to spiritual accompaniment.[46]

Catholic parents facing the shock of the NICU may be unfamiliar with the practice of neonatal palliative care. They should be counseled that it is deeply consistent with the Catholic tradition.

Care for the Dead: Burial, Autopsies, and Organ Donation

A brief word about Catholic teaching regarding care for the dead is worth including here. As noted previously, the protection and promotion of the dignity of neonatal patients is central to the Catholic tradition. At all times, the bodies of such patients—perinatal, living, dying, or dead—should be treated with the respect accorded all human persons. Roman Catholic canon law recommends that the remains of deceased persons be buried, although cremation is not prohibited.[47] The *Catechism* teaches that the bodies of the dead must be treated with respect and charity, noting the burial of the dead as one of the corporal works of mercy.[48] Such respectful treatment extends to fetal remains, whether the result of intentional abortion, miscarriage, or some other form of premature fetal demise. As Catholic ethicist Ron Hamel makes clear, fetal remains should never be considered or treated merely as medical waste.[49] In addition, as he notes:

> Also of great importance is the pastoral care of the parents who have experienced a tragic loss. As part of this care, parents should normally be the ones to arrange for the disposition of the remains of their fetus. If, for some reason, the parents are not able to do this, the hospital should then arrange for disposition, carefully informing the family of the hospital's procedures and ensuring that the family is comfortable with them.[50]

Hamel also provides a model policy on how to deal with fetal demise due to miscarriage or stillbirth.[51]

A related question is that of autopsy. Especially in complex neonatal cases, an autopsy may be warranted to determine an actual cause of death, or a particular infant may help advance the scientific understanding of her or his specific condition. Again, autopsies, respectfully done, are consistent with Catholic teaching. As the *Catechism* states: "Autopsies can be morally permitted for legal inquests or scientific research."[52]

Equally, organ donation and transplantation are supported by Catholic teaching. This is noted in both the *Catechism* (§2301) and the *ERDs*:

> Catholic health care institutions should encourage and provide the means whereby those who wish to do so may arrange for the donation of their organs and bodily tissue, for ethically legitimate purposes, so that they may be used for donation and research after death.
>
> Such organs should not be removed until it has been medically determined that the patient has died. In order to prevent any conflict of interest, the physician who determines death should not be a member of the transplant team.
>
> The use of tissue or organs from an infant may be permitted after death has been determined and with the informed consent of the parents or guardians.[53]

Thus, although autopsies and organ donation may not be the norm in most neonatal contexts, the Catholic tradition finds both to be acceptable practices as long as parental consent is obtained and the deceased infant is treated with the respect accorded a person with dignity.

Catholic Practices and Neonatal Care

While the teachings of the Catholic tradition shape many Catholic patients and families as they face medical crises, it is the case that, frequently, many Catholics are not familiar with the intricacies and nuances of Catholic teaching. Most Catholics, however, even—and sometimes, especially—lapsed Catholics are deeply familiar with the sacraments and sacramental practices of the Catholic tradition. These practices, often learned at a young age and learned in embodied and community-based ways over a lifetime, can have a more powerful effect on Catholic patients and families. How parents proceed with regard to medical decisions surrounding their infant children may, in the end, not be a matter so much of *what* is to be done medically but *how* it is done—not so much a matter of *what* decision is made but *how* they and their children are treated by the hospital and staff.

Practices and gestures that recognize parents and children as valued, relational beings are critical. And the ability for families to incorporate religious practices into the care of their imperiled children should be encouraged. Not only is this a matter of good patient care, but also allowing families to embed their children and the issues raised in their care in a larger framework shaped by ritual and sacrament may facilitate decision-making processes. In the final sections of this chapter, I would like to briefly discuss four key Catholic practices relevant to the neonatal context: baptism, anointing of the sick, prayers and blessings, and practices surrounding bereavement and funerals.

Baptism

The Catholic tradition endorses general good practice: that parents' understanding of their neonates as their children, as members of their family, as small *persons* with dignity requiring love and care should be recognized and nurtured at all times by healthcare staff. As with full-term healthy babies, parents should at all times and places be supported in their requests to see and hold and be present with their baby and should be offered opportunities to create identities and memories, even in the NICU. The bodies of babies—living or dead—should be treated with respect at all times.

More specifically, the Catholic tradition provides specific resources to families that if done well can help parents form their consciences. Baptism, for example, is an appropriate practice for all live-born babies, regardless of age, birth weight, or medical condition. Baptism affirms the sanctity and dignity of the infant—inviting the child into full membership in the Church regardless of illness or disability. But it also affirms the reality of death—for in baptism, Christians are baptized into the death of Christ. Granted, this is not usually emphasized during most baptismal ceremonies, but when performed well, the rite should equally emphasize reality and hope and should provide a spiritual and conceptual framework for the possibility that their child may be overmastered by their condition. When a priest or deacon is not available, anyone (even a nonbaptized person) may baptize with the consent of the parents.[54]

The issue of baptism for children who are stillborn or have died is a sensitive one. Canonically, the Catholic Church prohibits the baptism of those who have already died. For parents who wish baptism for their deceased child, a sensitive medical and pastoral staff should craft a middle ground event that encompasses all parties—including, perhaps, but not limited to, renewal of baptismal promises for the parents, the blessing and commendation of the child, and the blessing and commendation of the healthcare staff.

Anointing of the Sick

The Sacrament of the Anointing of the Sick is another potential practice with application to the neonatal context. Thoroughly revised after the Second Vatican Council forty years ago, the new understanding of the Sacrament of Anointing of the Sick (formerly Extreme Unction, which was reserved only for the dying) sees the rite as one *for the sick*. It entails anointing with blessed oil and laying on of hands together with prayers for healing and strength. In many ways, the practice of the Sacrament is in flux. Again, the Canon Law of the Church limits the Sacrament of Anointing to those baptized Catholics, gravely ill, who have "reached the age of reason," which is generally interpreted to be around six or seven years old. Other traditions akin to Roman Catholicism—including Orthodox Christianity and Eastern Catholic rites—do not have this limitation. And in pastoral practice, priests will often perform the Sacrament for sick children and their families. In instances where a priest will not anoint a child, there are many prayers that can be drawn from the rite (formally entitled *Pastoral Care of the Sick*), and more general ceremonies of prayer and blessing for the child, family, and caregivers can be developed.[55]

Like baptism, the Sacrament of the Sick practiced in the neonatal context should help family discernment by not shying away from the realities of grave illness and the real possibility of death while also reminding parents and caregivers that grace will surround their child both in death and in life. Both baptism and anointing also value, in important ways, the bodies of neonates, affirming the goodness of their bodies, even with pain, disability, and multiple medical interventions.

Prayers and Blessings

At all times, making space for ongoing prayer and blessings in the NICU, for and with the babies and families, is deeply consistent with the Catholic tradition. Rosaries, prayer cards, pictures of Our Lady of Guadalupe—the myriad aspects of material, religious culture—can be deeply sustaining to parents navigating the often frightening, uncomfortable, and intimidating environment of the NICU. These are especially important for parents from immigrant or ethnic communities for whom the US hospital may be particularly foreign and frightening. The rite of the *Pastoral Care for the Sick* includes a number of prayers and blessings for the sick, including a Blessing for Sick Children, which can be used by anyone at any time a blessing seems called for.[56]

Bereavement and Funerals

Attending to bereavement and mourning for parents who experience the death of a child in the neonatal context is extremely important. Many studies report that parents who experience perinatal death—late-term pregnancy loss, stillbirth, or infant death within the first month—find themselves bereft of many of the usual material social supports that normally would be provided to individuals in the case of a "real" birth or death.[57] Portraits of the ways that healthcare professional behave in instances of perinatal death are often quite unflattering.

In cases of perinatal death, the treatment of parents, the babies' bodies, and the parent–child bond should be attended to very intentionally. Again, parents should be supported in their requests to hold their dead child. Babies should not be taken to the mortuary until the parents are ready. Parents should be supported in their wish to take the baby home with them and to arrange for funeral services.

Pastoral ministers will find many resources in the Order of Christian Funerals, particularly Part II, "Funeral Rites for Children."[58] Some rites can be celebrated in the hospital or in the family home even if the child's body is not present— including "Prayers after Death," "Gathering in the Presence of the Body," or "Order for Blessing of Parents after a Miscarriage." Particularly suited to stillbirths and infants who have died soon after birth is the "Rite of Final Commendation for an Infant."[59] It can be celebrated in the hospital with or without the presence of the child and can be adapted to suit the particular needs of the family.

The public, communal character of Catholic liturgical rites is best respected when family, friends, and hospital staff are invited to participate both in rituals performed in the hospital and those performed in parishes. Such public acknowledgment can help address complications of perinatal grieving. The importance of the presence of members of the healthcare team at these events cannot be overstated.

Conclusion

The Catholic tradition provides a rich array of convictions, tradition, and practices that have formed parents who will walk into hospital NICUs and that can help them make informed decisions about treatment options for their children. Catholics will inhabit this tradition differently—there is no question about that. Many Catholics do not know their own tradition very well, or some may misinterpret it. And although the Roman Catholic tradition provides a relatively clear framework for reasoning about utilizing or withholding treatment, the application of that framework to specific cases is always more of an art than a science—even for those who know the tradition well.

In the end, although so much more could be said, I hope this chapter has conveyed that Catholicism is a tradition with a deep commitment to each and every person, regardless of disability; that it is a tradition that values the exercise of reason within the context of faith and spirituality; and that through prayer and sacramental practice, it seeks to create and sustain communities of persons in body, mind, and spirit—communities that encompass not only infants and their parents but also the wider circle of healthcare providers and caregivers who find themselves thrown together—often by surprise, often by tragedy—in the neonatal context.

Notes

1. Margaret E. Mohrmann, *Medicine as Ministry: Reflections on Suffering, Ethics, and Hope* (Cleveland, OH: Pilgrim, 1995).
2. Exodus 20:2-3 and Deuteronomy 5:6-7.
3. See William F. May, *The Physician's Covenant: Images of the Healer in Medical Ethics*, 2nd edition (Louisville, KY: Westminster John Knox, 2000), 30–35.
4. Mohrmann, 13.
5. Only two books have been published by Roman Catholic authors on neonatal medicine: Richard C. Sparks, *To Treat or Not to Treat: Bioethics and the Handicapped Newborn* (Mahwah, NJ: Paulist, 1988); and Charles C. Camosy, *Too Expensive to Treat? Finitude, Tragedy and the Neonatal ICU* (Grand Rapids, MI: Wm B. Eerdmans, 2010). The number of articles on neonatal medicine listed in the Catholic Periodical and Literature Index—the main research database for Catholic publications—over the past forty years can be counted on one hand.

6. Michael Lipka, "A Closer Look at Catholic America," Pew Research Center (September 15, 2015), accessed June 20, 2016, http://www.pewresearch.org/fact-tank/2015/09/14/a-closer-look-at-catholic-america/.

7. *The Catechism of the Catholic Church* (Mass Market Paperback, 1995), §§2383–85. The *Catechism of the Catholic Church* can be found on the Vatican website at: http://www.vatican.va/archive/ENG0015/_INDEX.HTM.

8. "'Catholics stand out with only 28% of the ever-married having divorced at some point' [compared with] . . . the 40% divorce rate for those with no religious affiliation, 39% for Protestants and 35% for those of other religious faiths. Overall, 26% of all American adults have divorced, whereas 20% of Catholics have done so." Wayne Laugesen, "Divorce Statistics Indicate Catholic Couples Are Less Likely to Break Up," *National Catholic Register* (November 14, 2013), accessed June 20, 2016, http://www.ncregister.com/daily-news/divorce-statistics-indicate-catholic-couples-are-less-likely-to-break-up/.

9. According to one source, "37% of women obtaining abortions identify themselves as Protestant, and 28% identify themselves as Catholic." "U.S. Abortion Statistics," Abort73.com (June 21, 2013), accessed June 20, 2016, http://www.abort73.com/abortion_facts/us_abortion_statistics/.

10. Michael Lipka, "Majority of U.S. Catholics' Opinions Run Counter to Church on Contraception, Homosexuality," *Pew Research Center* (September 19, 2013), accessed June 20, 2016, http://www.pewresearch.org/fact-tank/2013/09/19/majority-of-u-s-catholics-opinions-run-counter-to-church-on-contraception-homosexuality/.

11. Pew Research Center, "U.S. Catholics View Pope Francis as a Change for the Better," (March 6, 2014), accessed June 20, 2016, http://www.pewforum.org/2014/03/06/catholics-view-pope-francis-as-a-change-for-the-better/.

12. US Conference of Catholic Bishops, *The Ethical and Religious Directives for Catholic Health Care Services*, 6th edition, 2018. Henceforth abbreviated *ERDs*.

13. The notion of the dignity of the human person has been a staple of the Roman Catholic tradition throughout the twentieth century and has become increasingly central to Roman Catholic moral thought since the Second Vatican Council forward. It has also become a central concept in secular bioethics. In both traditions, it is more often simply asserted rather than defined, often precipitating confusion and masking the source of disagreements. In the Catholic tradition, the term is used to indicate that each human person—from a zygote to a person in a coma or with dementia at the end of life—is a being of inestimable value and transcendent, incomparable worth. Insofar as each human person bears the image of God, all human beings are to be inviolable. Regardless of capacities or health status, they are loved unconditionally and completely by God and are therefore to be loved unconditionally and completely by us. The concept applies not only in bioethics but also across the spectrum—social ethics, economic ethics, and so on.

For more on dignity in Catholic bioethics, see the encyclicals of John Paul II, *Evangelium Vitae*, nos. 2 and 96; Benedict XVI, Dignitatis *Personae*, no. 7; Francis, *Evangelii Gaudium*, no. 178; and Benedict XVI, *Caritas in Veritate*, no. 45. For a more extensive discussion of the topic within Roman Catholic bioethics, see, for just two examples, B. Andrew Lustig, "The Image of God and Human Dignity: A Complex Conversation," *Christian Bioethics* 23, no. 3 (December 2017): 317–34; and Edmund D. Pellegrino and Adam Schulman, *Human Dignity and Bioethics* (Notre Dame, IN: University of Notre Dame Press, 2009). For insight into the secular conversation, see, e.g., Leon Kass, *Life, Liberty, and the Defense of Dignity: The Challenge for Bioethics* (New York: Encounter Books, 2002).

14. *ERDs*, p. 10. The dignity of the human person is mentioned twenty-one times in the thirty-eight pamphlet-sized pages of the *ERDs*, beginning in the Preamble and informing every subsection except the section on the formation of partnerships between hospitals and health systems (though it is presumed there as well).

15. See Catholics for Choice website, accessed June 20, 2016, http://www.catholicsforchoice.org/abortion/.

16. Some Catholic theologians have based their argument for the personhood of embryos and fetuses on their inherent *potential* to exercise certain capacities. Other theologians have argued that embryos do not become persons until implantation prevents twinning, thus establishing an *individual*. For the most comprehensive overview of these positions, see Michael R. Panicola, "Three Views on the Preimplantation Embryo," *National Catholic Bioethics Quarterly* 2, no. 1 (Spring 2002): 69–97. The positions outlined by Panicola are not well known by Catholic lay persons and are not the official position of the Catholic Church.

17. At issue in one of the seminal cases in neonatal medicine and ethics—the Baby Doe case—was a perception by the medical staff that Baby Doe was not treated respectfully, as a person with dignity. Denied surgical treatment and nutrition and hydration due to his Down syndrome, Baby Doe was largely moved to the side and allowed to die. See Allen Verhey, "The Death of Infant Doe: Jesus and the Neonates," in *On Moral Medicine: Theological Perspectives on Medical Ethics*, 3rd edition, ed. M. Therese Lysaught and Joseph Kotva (Grand Rapids, MI: Wm B. Eerdmans, 2012), 796–800.

18. *ERDs*, p. 18.

19. *ERDs*, Directives 27 and 28.

20. *Gaudium et Spes*, The Pastoral Constitution on the Church in the Modern World, number 16; see also the *Catechism of the Catholic Church*, §1776–1802.

21. Importantly, the discussion of conscience within the *Catechism of the Catholic Church* is located under the larger subheading of "The Dignity of the Human Person."

22. *ERDs*, Directives 56 and 57.

23. Pius XII, "Address to an International Congress of Anesthesiologists," November 24, 1957.

24. As the *ERDs* state: "We have a duty to preserve our life and to use it for the glory of God, but the duty to preserve life is not absolute, for we may reject life-prolonging procedures that are insufficiently beneficial or excessively burdensome" (p. 29).

25. Congregation for the Doctrine of the Faith, *Declaration on Euthanasia*, 1980.

26. *Catechism*, §2278.

27. *Catechism*, §2276.

28. See Ronald Hamel and James Walters, *Artificial Nutrition and Hydration and the Permanently Unconscious Patient: The Catholic Debate* (Washington,

DC: Georgetown University Press, 2007); and Christopher Tollefsen, ed. *Artificial Nutrition and Hydration: The New Catholic Debate* (Dordrecht: Springer, 2010).

29. "Address of John Paul II to the Participants in the International Congress on 'Life-Sustaining Treatments and Vegetative State: Scientific Advances and Ethical Dilemmas," 2004.

30. *ERDs*, Directive 58.

31. *Catechism*, §2276.

32. Congregation for the Doctrine of the Faith, *Declaration on Euthanasia*, 1980, Part II.

33. John Paul II, *Evangelium Vitae*, 1995, §12.

34. Ibid., §19.

35. *ERDs*, Directive 3.

36. See James F. Drane, "Anencephaly and the Interruption of Pregnancy: Policy Proposals for HECs," *HEC Forum* 4, no. 2 (1992): 103–19; James L. Walsh and Moira M. McQueen, "The Morality of Induced Delivery of the Anencephalic Fetus prior to Viability," *Kennedy Institute of Ethics Journal* 3, no. 4 (1993): 357–69; Kevin O'Rourke and Jean deBlois, "Induced Delivery of Anencephalic Fetuses: A Response to James L. Walsh and Moira M. McQueen," *Kennedy Institute of Ethics Journal* 4, no. 1 (1994): 47–53; and Kevin O'Rourke, "Ethical Opinions in Regard to the Question of Early Delivery of Anencephalic Infants," *Linacre Quarterly* 63, no. 3 (1996): 55–59.

37. National Conference of Catholic Bishops, Doctrine Committee, "Moral Principles Concerning Infants with Anencephaly," *Origins* 26, no. 17 (October 10, 1996).

38. See, e.g., Ira Byock, *The Best Care Possible: A Physician's Quest to Transform Care through the End of Life* (New York: Avery, 2013).

39. For those not familiar with the WHO definition, it states: "Palliative care is an approach that improves the quality of life of patients and their families facing the problem associated with life-threatening illness, through the prevention and relief of suffering by means of early identification and impeccable assessment and treatment of pain and other problems, physical, psychosocial and spiritual. Palliative care: provides relief from pain and other distressing symptoms; affirms life and regards dying as a normal process; intends neither to hasten or postpone death; integrates the psychological and spiritual aspects of patient care; offers a support system to help patients live as actively as possible until death; offers a support system to help the family cope during the patients' illness and in their own bereavement; uses a team approach to address the needs of patients and their families, including bereavement counseling, if indicated; will enhance quality of life, and may also positively influence the course of illness; and is applicable early in the course of illness, in conjunction with other therapies that are intended to prolong life, such as chemotherapy or radiation therapy, and includes those investigations needed to better understand and manage distressing clinical complications." See: http://www.who.int/cancer/palliative/definition/en/.

40. Ibid.

41. See, e.g., Romanus Cessario, O.P., "Catholic Considerations on Palliative Care," *National Catholic Bioethics Quarterly* (Winter 2006): 639–50; and Suzanne Gross, F.S.E., and Marie T. Hilliard, R.N., "Palliative Care, Pain Management, and Human Suffering," in *Catholic Health Care Ethics: A Manual for Practitioners*, ed. Edward J. Furton with Peter J. Cataldo and Albert S. Moraczewski, O.P. (Philadelphia: National Catholic Bioethics Center, 2009), 193–97.

42. See, e.g., Ronald Hamel, "Palliative Care Needs a Culture to Sustain It," *Health Progress* (January–February 2011): 70–72; Tina Picchi, "Palliative Care: A Hallmark of Catholic Mission," *Health Progress* (January–February 2011): 11; and "How Four Systems Approach Palliative Care," *Health Progress* (January–February 2011): 27–37.

43. *Catechism*, §2279.

44. Benedict XVI, "For the Fifteenth World Day of the Sick," December 8, 2006.

45. Ibid.

46. Benedict XVI, "Meeting with the Authorities and the Diplomatic Corps [Austria]," September 7, 2007. Or, as he stated in his address to healthcare workers in November 2007: "Indeed, recourse to the use of palliative care when necessary is correct, which, even though it cannot heal, can relieve the pain caused by illness. Alongside the in-dispensable clinical treatment, however, it is always necessary to show a concrete capacity to love, because the sick need understanding, comfort and constant encour-agement and accompaniment" (Benedict XVI, "Address of His Holiness Benedict XVI to the 22nd International Congress of the Pontifical Council for Health Pastoral Care," November 17, 2007).

47. *Code of Canon Law*, Book IV, Part II, Title III, Canon 1176, §3.

48. Catechism, §2300.

49. Ron Hamel, "Some Guidance on Disposition of Fetal Remains," *Health Care Ethics USA* (Spring 2008): 8–9.

50. Ibid., 9.

51. Ibid., 10.

52. *Catechism*, §2301.

53. *ERDs*, Directives 63–65.

54. As it states in *The Catechism of the Catholic Church*, §1256: "The ordinary ministers of Baptism are the bishop and priest and, in the Latin Church, also the deacon. In case of necessity, anyone, even a non-baptized person, with the required intention, can baptize, by using the Trinitarian baptismal formula. The intention required is to will to do what the Church does when she baptizes. The Church finds the reason for this possibility in the universal saving will of God and the necessity of Baptism for salvation."

55. *Pastoral Care of the Sick: Rites of Anointing and Viaticum* (Collegeville, MN: Liturgical Press, 1983).

56. Examples of these prayers and blessings can be found on the website of the US Conference of Catholic Bishops, "Order for the Blessing of the Sick," accessed June

20, 2016, http://www.usccb.org/prayer-and-worship/sacraments-and-sacramentals/sacramentals-blessings/persons/order-for-the-blessing-of-the-sick.cfm.

57. Claudia Malacrida, "Complicating Mourning: The Social Economy of Perinatal Death," *Qualitative Health Research* 9, no. 4 (July 1999): 504–19.

58. *Order of Christian Funerals with Cremation Rite* (Totowa, NJ: Catholic Book Publishing, 1990).

59. Ibid., §§337–42.

3

Reading Tragedy through the Christian Story

An Anabaptist Perspective

Erin Dufault-Hunter

Unlike with my own high-risk pregnancy due to age, Paul and Susan were a young and healthy couple in our church small group. When Susan became pregnant with their first child, we did all the usual celebrating that marks such announcements and offered thanks for new life. But during a routine visit to the doctor in the second trimester, their newly-minted obstetrician-gynecologist saw something unusual on the ultrasound and decided to send them to a local imaging center for a detailed scan. Glancing at Susan lying on the table, a gruff but highly competent doctor delivered the news: the fetus had a serious abnormality, which the amniocentesis would soon confirm as Trisomy 13.[1] Thus began their unexpected journey as parents of a child with a limited future.

Because their family, congregation, and healthcare providers cooperated to sustain these friends with honesty and grace, this tragic story of a dying infant also became an occasion of beauty and costly hope. His short life pressed all of us to face the poignant, aching fragility of life and to recognize the power of bearing witness to sorrow. In his dying, those who worship the Christian God had to ask how our faith mattered amid such anguish, and we will explore in the following pages how this faith shaped how they made decisions about both medical and nonmedical care for their son. As a key caveat, whenever they tell their story, Paul and Susan insist that others' willingness to accompany them made possible their choices and particular path of parenting a dying infant. They are aware that many face similar diagnoses or other tragedies without resources that make the burden of grief bearable.

In the context of medicine, it is not only parents of children with serious disorders who require such resources for bearing sorrow. We know that grief comes to all of us, unbeckoned and unwelcome. But those engaged in health care stand in a unique position in that they are regularly exposed to heart-wrenching circumstances, and those encountered in labor and delivery or neonatal intensive care are some of the most shattering. This essay assumes that by its very nature, grief demands our attention; however much we wish to ignore it, heartache insists on expression. Thus, healthcare providers must attend to their sorrows, regardless of whether they arise from their personal life or in their professional context. By intentionally developing practices of mourning, nurses and doctors can be present to parents in the ways demanded by care, rather than driven by their own accumulated (conscious or unconscious) heartbreak.

In this essay, I reflect on parents' experience of giving birth to dead or dying children and caregivers' tending of these families as interpreted through an Anabaptist, evangelical Christian faith.[2] One way of explaining "evangelical" faith is that we are Christians who claim the Bible and, more specifically, the story of Jesus in a way that it becomes our own story; that is, we seek to read our own lives filtered through this text. At the heart of that Scriptural drama for us is the cross, a sign that claims, among other things, that the goodness and power of God redeems anguish. While God often fails to do this in ways clearly evident to us, we trust that the Spirit enters into our sadness, preventing sorrow from having the last word.

By exploring stories of the heartbreak that dying or stillborn babies evoke, I hope not only to explain evangelical Mennonite beliefs but to also display how such faith shaped our responses to tragedy. I offer these reflections as a gift to both encourage and challenge healthcare providers in neonatal contexts. First, I hope to inspire medical professionals to engage with coming alongside them as parents access their faith and, when possible, enabling them to attach to their infant with a limited future. In doing so, healthcare providers collaborate with families of faith to create sacred spaces even in the valley of the shadow of death.[3] When caregivers mix straightforwardness about the prognosis with sensitivity to parents' need for lament, they help foster an environment in which Christians can enact a costly hope in the resurrection. But I also offer these thoughts as a gift that is simultaneously a challenge to medical personnel, pressing them to attend to their own grief. Defying our efforts to ignore it, the emotion of grief refuses to be neglected and instead can arise unheeded to choke out compassionate care. Because of the nature of grief and of their profession, providers who practice mourning are also empowered to extend the gracious presence necessary for true patient care, especially amid the sorrow and tender beauty that characterize the neonatal context.

Ordinary Practices in an Extraordinary Time: Trisomy and Faithful Parenting

For the devout, faith provides a narrative not only for making meaning in some theoretical sense but also for establishing patterns of everyday life. The couple mentioned previously—Paul and Susan—were members of our small Mennonite congregation, and they had intentionally developed habits informed by our faith.[4] As Mennonites, we interpret our lives as those baptized into a broader stream of the Christian tradition called Anabaptist; we trust that Scripture truthfully witnesses to God and guides us into wholeness or what is often called "salvation."[5] Without going into nuances of doctrine or Biblical interpretation, our way of telling the Christian story assumes at least the following: the God who created all that exists came to us in Jesus to show humans how we are meant to live; God offers us help in such living through the Spirit who dwells with us; this same Spirit provides guidance through Scripture and especially through mutual discernment within the community of faith. Some major characteristics of our tradition include commitments to simplicity and justice, with hospitality as a core value. Another main trait is the commitment to nonviolence, a commitment rooted among other things in our confidence that God's love will ultimately right the world. We hold the belief common among Christians (but surely a rather bizarre one to many, especially in our scientific age) in God's resurrection of our bodies. These last two specific tenets underscore the overarching sense shared by devout Christians across traditions that we are not ultimately in charge of our own lives, and thus faith means actively trusting Christ in every aspect of our lives. Importantly regarding infants, Mennonites do not believe in "original sin" (i.e., that babies are born in a state of sin); we dedicate children until they reach an age when they choose to follow Jesus and be baptized—or they choose not to.

Most of the time, we muddle along in our lives, worshipping and working in mundane and ordinary ways. But then come moments like the one Susan encountered on that exam table, when a new reality explodes our expectations and dreams; even otherwise ordinary things become poignant or painful. These moments often raise questions about why or how our faith matters, especially when material conditions—such as the imminent death of our infant child—do not change. Until that point, Susan had plotted her life along another narrative of childbearing in which babies are put together rightly, chromosomes pair correctly, and bodies form with major systems intact. In North America, we often expect to give birth to healthy children aided by effective medical help. But when Paul and Susan heard that their baby—a son—was severely deformed, disabled, and unlikely to survive to term, they lacked a ready script. Susan and Paul had to reconsider what parenting this little boy meant and ponder how they would actively welcome a child with a limited future into a womb rather than resent the way his brokenness shattered the usual pattern of "what to expect when you're expecting." Family and community wondered how to come alongside them in the tenuous reality of Trisomy, some of us barely holding back fears or memories this pregnancy raised for us.

For those who, like us, believe that God is implicated in every aspect of our lives, we now had to determine how to enact the Christian story amid this distress. To do this required improvisation (i.e., thinking and acting in new ways) that was also bounded by long-standing beliefs encoded in patterns of living. From the moment of diagnosis onward, customary parental patterns raised questions and rubbed my friends' emotions raw. To grasp how Christian faith shaped these parents' lives, I explore in this chapter how this couple and our community reimagined parenting. I also note how, occasionally, medical professionals ably came alongside them in their journey, enabling them to live faithfully amid the disruption such heartbreak brings.

Unfortunately, the physician who did the preliminary imaging broke the news of the grave disorder with little compassion. Given the brusque, insensitive manner of the doctor, other medical staff at the clinic quickly swept my stunned friends into a counseling room. The staff person began by gently offering the possibility of terminating the pregnancy. Tellingly, neither Susan nor Paul entertained this option, and they did not "make a decision" not to terminate. Raised within their particular faith community and within a tradition that sustained people amid pain, this was a path simply unavailable to them, akin to an act of violence that pacifism forbade them. When they tell this part of their story, they quickly note that unlike many who face such circumstances, they knew that family and friends would concretely support their family, whatever their future held. (Susan and Paul do not see themselves as particularly courageous or exemplary; however painful things were, their strong web of relationships made facing an unknown future with a Trisomy infant possible. They recognize as much as anyone why others choose other paths.) The counselor changed tack, and she gently offered them an overview of the condition, statistics, and treatment. They left the office, and, as highly educated adults in our Internet era, they began to study this disorder called Trisomy 13.

From this point forward, Paul and Susan accessed medical care, open-eyed to the prognosis of their boy while seeking to enact their faith. Crucially, once their ob-gyn understood that faith and medical facts would inform their approach to the pregnancy, she offered clear information, not sugar-coating expectations or physical realities, yet did so with kindness and attentiveness. While some doctors might have struggled to extend space to these young parents to explore the intersection of their convictions with harsh biological realities, their primary caregiver throughout this ordeal never wavered in her willingness to join them in their journey as their doctor. Having begun their journey in shock and disorientation at the imaging center, Susan and Paul now sought a new course for how to be faithful Christian parents to their son.

The next season of bearing a profoundly disabled fetus brought unforeseen challenges, which were made more poignant by the seemingly endless encounter of seemingly ordinary things made sharp and painful by their son's condition. For example, Susan recalls the custom of strangers commenting to pregnant women, making polite conversation or seeking connection by asking about due dates or sharing woes about the discomfort of expecting. But of course what Susan "expected" did not make for polite conversation, and she constantly had to decide how to be kind to people whose comments unknowingly sliced her to the core—usually graciously abstaining from pushing on them a truth that would pain them in turn, such as, "My child is deformed and disabled and probably will die before birth."

Given that their son might die in utero and given such chronic reminders of her own (and perhaps her son's) pain, Susan began to pray for his death to come quickly. While waiting for most pregnant couples is expectation, Paul and Susan found the waiting—waiting for him to die, waiting for him to come to term—excruciating. In response to the daily brutality of lingering in this physical and emotional space, an artist in our church designed a beautiful clock face for them. Hours corresponded to dates, and for each date, different members of our community offered them gifts (e.g., dinners, tickets to movies, activities) to ease the burden that waiting placed on them. The clock itself witnessed to our willingness to stand with them under the oppressive, uncontrollable weight of time.

Despite our prayers for a miscarriage, this little boy continued to live and grow inside Susan. As the weeks stretched on, she talked with an aunt who was not only a Mennonite but also an experienced nurse. In the conversation, she gently encouraged Susan to dare to hope for something else, for a pregnancy that came to term. Despite the multiple difficulties of this, her aunt noted that in her experience, the opportunity for parents to actually hold their baby—to have the chance to say goodbye—had helped many of them—especially mothers—with their grief. As a daughter of a therapist and as someone being trained as one, this made sense to Susan. Now their prayers and those who came alongside them shifted course again, and we pleaded for the boy to live long enough for such a meeting. Again, their ob-gyn supported them as they discerned each step, offering a kind presence combined with good care—a grace whose value was impossible to measure during such a stressful and anxious time.

I noted earlier that cases such as Trisomy 13 cause Christians to reconsider otherwise ordinary patterns, practices, or beliefs about babies. In this instance, these came together in unexpected ways when a common assertion about children was mixed with an otherwise exciting or fun parental responsibility. The glibly stated claim—shared by many, regardless of faith—is that children are a gift; the usually intense but joyful parental practice is the privilege of naming our children. Susan and Paul determined that they needed to bind themselves to their son by naming him in this waiting season, a concrete way to welcome him amid the uncertainty of Trisomy. Having served as missionaries together in Eastern Europe, they gave him an English name and a Lithuanian one, so his surname translated to, "Gift given by God." Then as many Christians do when seeking counsel, they came to our pastor, a man who worked not only as a minister but also as a Hebrew Bible ("Old Testament") scholar. They told him their son's name (abbreviated here as "N.D." for confidentiality) and what it meant. Then, in an act of defiance, faith, and doubt rolled into one, they challenged him: "Now, tell us how this can be true." How could this broken fetus—perhaps even a suffering one—be a gift?

Our pastor had performed many baby dedications (including those of my own children). In that ceremony, we offer thanksgiving and bless them. But we also do something else: we offer the child back to God, vowing that we will train our children for faithfulness, no matter what that might mean. We do this in a tradition that recalls the bloody martyrdom of many of our foreparents. (Mennonites were tortured and killed because of their stance toward the state and their pacifism, and some of these early stories are collected in *The Martyr's Mirror*, a book found on many of our bookshelves.) Most important, the explicit recognition that they belong to God reminds us to loosen our grip on our children—children we want to both control and protect. But, for Christians, parenthood is not our own story to tell; rather, it is a role we enact within God's larger, overarching drama. Our pastor had also cut his theological teeth on the Old Testament. In that diverse collection of stories and poems, the main character YHWH (or "the LORD") created all that is and abounds in steadfast love toward this creation yet cannot be manipulated or controlled by the human beings made to worship and to partner with him.[6]

Our minister's reply to "How is this true?" relied on this vision of God and this same God's power to raise Jesus from the dead. In summary, he replied to my friends, "Perhaps N.D. is primarily a gift to God—not to you." On the face of it, this sounds callous or smacks against the sentimentality that surrounds parenting in our culture, a sentimentality that also makes bearing dead, chronically ill, or dying children problematic, to say the least. Our pastor is a kind man. Yet, as a minister, he took seriously the notion that, much as a doctor needs to speak honestly about "what is" or what we know medically, a minister needs to truthfully recall "what is" or what we know from within the Christian story. Thus, he pressed Susan and Paul (and all of us who accompanied them) to remember core convictions of our faith, a faith that makes sense only within a narrative of God's loving power to redeem tragedy for God's beloved. The pastor's synopsis shocked believers back to the very core of our faith. We do not determine how our children's lives before—and for—God will go; while we comfort and guide them as we can, we cannot protect them from all suffering. Instead, the God of the universe holds our lives and redeems our pain, finally by offering us a home with her eternally, raising us into new life as her children, servants, and friends. Our pastor's response pushed N.D.'s parents further into the Christian story, giving them the ability to act in a way that was consistent with their belief in their son's ultimate value as God's beloved.

This boy came to a particular community, one in which regular rituals remind us that we cannot always protect our children from pain (and thus not protect ourselves from suffering) as well as a tradition that tells stories of redemptive suffering. As a Trisomy infant, his arrival caused all of us to reconsider cultural and religious assumptions asserting that children are gifts to and for *us*. Basic orthodox Christian teaching claims that the world is God's; even our children belong to God, and so we surrender them to God's good care.[7] Much as moderns seek to avoid its reality or mask its presence through the wonder of medicine, death comes for all of us. While we Christians sometimes glibly affirm children as gifts and attest to the resurrection of the body, this little boy's life caused all of us to reconsider how radical such assumptions can be and how they intertwine to expose our core convictions about the nature of human existence and our hope amid reminders of mortality. Joined to our community by his broken body, we had to face the unsettling reality that not only this boy but all our children breathe by virtue of the gift of the One who puffed into Adam's muddy nostrils.[8] In so doing, this boy recalled our ultimate status as fragile, dependent creatures who nonetheless are made for joyful communion with God through the power of the resurrection.

As we prayed he would, the boy survived long enough to be born and to be born alive. In the moment of his birth and during his short life span, well-worn habits and core convictions again converged to inform this unusual circumstance. Susan and Paul asked the pastor, his wife, and their immediate family to be ready to come into the room after the cesarean delivery. There they engaged in the practice of baby dedication mentioned earlier, a ritual especially crucial for those Mennonites who do not baptize infants. Usually a happy affair celebrated in front of the entire congregation during a service, this boy's consecration took place in post-op. Anointed with oil by the minister, the boy was named and blessed, claimed as a member of our community while also pronounced as God's own child. As usually stated but in this context stripped of mere sentimentality, the parents released their son to the God who created him for herself; grandparents, uncles, and aunts acted on behalf of the entire church body, confirming this reality with sometimes sobbing "Amens."[9] Packed into a tiny hospital room, family members held this little baby as he struggled to breathe, cooing over him and wetting his face with their tears. Born with severe problems with his respiratory system, he died in his mother's arms three hours later.[10] (Years later when showing us pictures of him, she confessed that she had worried that his deformity might make it difficult to attach to him, but this fear proved unfounded—for her as for her entire family. I suspect that practices of intention-ally welcoming and actively waiting for him aided this.)

Despite the intimacy of the situation, not only family had piled into this room to witness to this little boy's life and to claim him as beloved. Naturally, the med-ical staff had had to be notified about the service and bend the rules a bit re-garding visitors; without such flexibility, bonding in this way through ceremony and presence in this sacred space would not have been possible. But when some of the medical staff heard of the plans for a service of dedication, they timidly requested if, pending other patient needs, they could attend. While one certainly hopes for compassion among all healthcare providers, I affectionately refer to medical staff in specialties such as the neonatal intensive care unit (NICU) and labor and delivery as "mushballs." Committed to the welfare of their patients and families, they also tend to be deeply affected by their stories. Here was a tale tinged with sorrow but also with something else—perhaps with a costly hope—which several of the hospital staff found alluring. Given that hospitality is a core value for Mennonites, it was natural that my friends accepted their request, extending an intimate circle to encompass those who too seldom get the oppor-tunity to come alongside families in this way.

One of the staff remarked to the parents before they left the hospital, "I think that boy was loved more in three hours than many children are in a lifetime." Such a statement could be unpacked in a variety of ways, but here I will briefly make two observations. First, one cannot underestimate the value of the staff's willingness to secure time and space for this gathering. It indicates how crucial cooperation and adaptability in hospital settings can be for people of faith, espe-cially when such rituals require a community to witness to it. Second, "love" of their Trisomy son did not translate for these parents into "doing all they could" to keep him alive for however long they could do so. With core convictions about the fragility of life and the presence of God in the midst of our pain, they fo-cused on being present to him in what they perceived as his suffering rather than seeking to alleviate it, and they risked the agony of loving attachment to an infant with a limited future. Many parents (including Christian ones) believe that val-uing their child's life means extending it at all costs, and I do not begrudge this impulse or its application under other conditions. Susan and Paul did not think about nonintervention in formal terms such as "futility"; nor was the choice due to his lack of worth. But as they researched and talked with medical staff about their son's probable condition at birth (as well as what was possible given tech-nology), they weighed this against their determination to simultaneously claim him and entrust him to God. To choose on other grounds than such perilous hospitality to this broken and beloved infant would have said more about their fear of death than about their love for him, more about their desire to stave off loss than about expressing faithfulness by joining their lives to a dying child.

Our tradition does recall the inevitability of tragedy in a fractured world, but it also exposes that there are much worse things than pain. In a tradition that honors martyrs and follows a crucified God, N.D.'s parents knew that the greatest suffering is not pain per se but rather the isolation that pain so often generates.[11] Thus, for however long he lived, they resolved to not abandon their son in his suffering. To come to this place required that they work with the hospital staff to determine the logistics of such joining, but they finally trusted not in medical intervention. Instead, they leaned into a Christ who is present to the afflicted and entrusted their family's story to his Spirit who, against the mysterious horizon of eternity, redeems tragedy so tenderly offered.

In addition, the nurse's comment about the family's love for N.D. exposes the emotional and psychological sensitivity of many who serve on NICU teams. They recognize the sorrow that lays like a shadow over some who come through their doors. This comment brings to our attention the dearth of resources we have for attending to grief—not only for Christians but also for healthcare providers. I suspect that the hospital staff wanted to attend this ceremony not merely for Susan, Paul, and their son's sake but rather for all the children and families to whose affliction they had borne witness, affliction they carried as practitioners in the wondrous yet vulnerable space of neonatal care. In the next section, I consider how medical staff in these contexts need to attend to their own sorrow so that they are free to facilitate healing in the ways displayed by the attentive staff that served Paul, Susan, their son, and his family.

Practitioners Playing Whack-a-Mole: Why Grief Must Become Mourning

My husband and I leaned against the hospital wall, his arms around me as we both quietly wept. From the room behind us came an explosion of wailing, sorrow finally released from the boundary that shock had provided. These friends had become miraculously, unexpectedly, even initially undesirably pregnant. But what could only be described as glee and giddiness quickly took over. Our community was overjoyed, taking delighted satisfaction in the disturbance of their planned lives, in contrast to many of us who had children. We threw showers and documented the pregnancy in cute pictures, and these friends experienced the joy of unexpected expectation.

But, without warning, their little girl died full-term, and because of distance, their family could not make it to the emergency cesarean delivery the day before. When the doctor confirmed her worst fears about the meaning of her daughter's sudden stillness, my friend had gone into shock. She spoke and acted without visible distress, blankly staring as she went through the horror of giving birth and then cradling her perfectly formed, dead infant. Now, with her parents' and sisters' arrival, the dam broke, and she wailed as sheer anguish required.

The medical staff had been kind, moving her as soon as possible out of labor and delivery and putting her in a room as far as possible from other patients. They placed a postcard with a dew-touched leaf to her door, a sign of her condition to other staff. The night before, labor and delivery personnel had bent hospital rules, arranging for close friends who had gathered to come in pairs into the post-op room. There, we held their daughter in short turns, blessing her and kissing her before turning her body over to her parents. Her mother and father held her for hours, until reluctantly they released her body to the morgue. As with Susan and Paul, we found the medical team remarkably sensitive to our situation, kindly facilitating our need to connect with this little girl and her parents. But in sharp contrast to our experience thus far, the lone woman sitting almost directly across from us at the nurse's station conveyed little compassion. Instead, she fidgeted and sighed obnoxiously, clearly irritated—and wanting us to know it.

After several minutes of this, she began saying to us and to no one in particular, "She needs to stop doing that. She needs to stop crying." I tensed up. While a Mennonite by conviction, I am not naturally nonviolent; knowing this, my husband instinctively tightened his grip around my waist. She continued to do this for several minutes, even taking the opportunity to chide my friend's sister, who had come to her desk to get more tissues. (Thankfully, she was too stunned by her tone and commands to do anything but give us a look of complete disbelief before returning to her sister.) The nurse continued undeterred, now adding another element to her demand for silence, saying, "She can have another one. She needs to stop doing that." In response to the rage this ignorant statement evoked in me, my husband clasped me more tightly, saying, "Down, mama bear." I whispered a promise to get a handle on my emotion, but I also vowed I would not allow this woman to spew these inane cruelties onto our friends.

Sufficiently convinced of my self-control, my husband eventually released me, and I walked over to her desk. As I approached, she began again, insisting that the crying needed to stop and that she could have another child. (This last statement was especially galling; their chances of conceiving had been so minuscule that their doctor had told them birth control was unnecessary.) I tried to interject amid her uncontrollable loop of comments, when suddenly she said it: "This happened to me." I felt my body slowly alter course, conscious that I needed to create space for something other than my anger. I took some deep breaths and then managed to ask her the question her revelation begged: "What happened to you?"

The nurse began to tell her story, revealing that she had given birth to not one but two dead children. Odd given her litany, she herself was never able to "have another one" and bore no other children. She came from a culture that practiced mourning, but her husband and her family had forbidden this, insisting that she move past these losses. And she had done that, she said, eventually adopting two boys. At this point her tenor altered, becoming less agitated. She seemed proud of her sons and very attached to them. Something caught my attention as she chattered about her boys and their sports teams. I inquired about their ages. The older boy was twelve and had been adopted near birth. I was stunned. This meant that the grief spilling out of her today was not from a fresh wound; rather, it arose from sorrows stuffed deeply inside her at least a decade and a half before. I listened for a bit longer, asking for some details about her sons, noticing how in her calmed state she now was speaking *with* me, rather than speaking *at* me.

Having exhausted her pent-up energy by engaging her in the narrative and noting that she was now able to converse with me, I turned the conversation back to the present. First, I told her how glad I was for her and for her boys. I then informed her that it was going to be okay; we are going to cry, I said, and "It will be all right." She initially protested a bit, beginning her earlier script against our tears but with less fervor. I repeated to her that we would be weeping and again reassured her, repeating the vague phrase, "It will be all right." I could not think of another way to honestly reflect the sliver of faith we had as we gave in to our sorrow. I thanked her for sharing her story and then returned to my husband, who soon would accompany the girl's father, dressing her for burial. The nurse settled in, never again commenting about our responses to this death.

"Blessed Are Those Who Mourn, for They Shall Be Comforted"

In the Gospel of Matthew, Jesus gives a series of blessings, some of them seemingly bizarre. One of the most unsettling for me had always been, "Blessed are those who mourn, for they shall be comforted."[12] It seemed to blithely celebrate sorrow, and as someone prone to being overwhelmed by sadness, this felt dangerous and far from good news. Listening to that nurse at the hospital, suddenly the penny dropped for me about this text. It does not praise loss or anguish itself. Rather, Jesus proclaims that those who practice mourning—those who engage in rituals of lament—are those who open themselves to God's comfort. As a theological ethicist, I take this to be true not merely for followers of Christ but for all of us, whatever our religious convictions (or lack thereof). Psychology might agree, framing this insight in therapeutic rather than religious language.

Whatever our academic discipline or authoritative source, many experience grief as a jealous emotion that relentlessly demands our attention. Unfortunately, like this nurse, we may be encouraged by our community or by our own fear to deny it, to stuff it inside ourselves as if we could lock such an emotion in a watertight capsule, stashed away so that it will not leak into other parts of our lives.

On the face of it, this seems necessary; we cannot imagine surviving the tsunami of sorrow that wells up in us at the loss of infants and children. Further, we suspect—sometimes rightly—that when we honestly reveal how profoundly we have been shattered, others (even intimates like spouses or family) will abandon us. Biological realities—from chromosomal abnormalities to diseases that inexplicably claim those we love—threaten people who work hard to maintain an illusion of control. For such persons, the inconsolability of honest anguish terrifies them. They retreat from us in our agony, refusing to be collateral damage to our grief's force. Yet, this withdrawal ultimately proves futile. Trying to ignore bereavement is like playing whack-a-mole: by its nature, grief refuses to remain hidden but instead pops up at another time and place—and never does so at our choosing.[13]

When grief demands our attention, we can weather its threatening brutality by engaging in practices of mourning. For our purposes, I distinguish between mourning (or lament) and grief, with the former an intentional response to the latter. Unlike other tempting reactions to sorrow such as retreat or denial, engaging in lament does not merely deflect grief (as if it cannot touch us); nor does mourning empower us to extinguish our anguish. Instead, mourning serves at least three purposes. First, mourning enables us to feel and express grief's impact without being utterly controlled or silenced by it; even if in the midst of it, survival against sorrow's intensity often feels precarious. Second, mourning weakens grief's capacity to shatter our relationships, to sever us from others as well as from ourselves. Last, lament expands the hearts of those who engage in it, creating space in us not only for others' sadness but also for their joy.

Like other professionals who regularly enter into vulnerable spaces in the course of their work, healthcare providers must consider how they will respond when grief enters, uninvited, into those places. The nurse's denial of grief illustrates how stifling grief causes it to gain strength over time, irrepressibly bubbling up to render such a caregiver deaf and blind to her patient and her needs. Our weeping lanced her sick heart, and out spewed the infection of a grief denied. Despite extensive training and despite her determination to repress it, this grief overtook the nurse's actions toward her patients. She appeared unaware of this takeover, as stifled heartache fractured not only her external relationships but also her relationship to herself, to her own body and soul that longed for sorrow's release. Finally, grief impaired her ability to be present and care for others, even her patients. Tellingly, our anguish sparked not a response of sadness or sympathy, which would seem logical. Rather, our weeping triggered anger, a resentment that we could release our grief while her own remained pent up inside her. Her response underscores the need for medical professionals to engage in rituals of mourning so that they release the pressure of their grief and attach to patients (and others) in a way that expands providers' capacity for compassionate care.

It may seem implausible to posit that healthcare providers must intentionally engage in mourning in order to be present to their patients or their families. Sometimes people speak as if medical personnel need to foster not connection but rather "professional distance." On one level, this makes sense, as they need to treat the (body of the) person in front of them and thus fulfill their obligation of (physical) care.[14] But as healthcare professionals know, the reality of grief often intersects with their work, sometimes catching them unprepared for what their witness to it costs them. The toll such presence can take on healthcare professionals came home to me one year while teaching my bioethics course.

For the final project, I invited students to respond to the material we had covered either by writing an academic paper or engaging in a creative art project. I realize that many of my students have experiences they best integrate with their faith through nonlinear, "right-brain" activities. One of the most surprising, impactful pieces submitted so far was a triptych (a three-paneled altar piece). Simple in construction and style, the triptych featured images that were arresting and unexpected. On the furthest left panel was a woman in scrubs, slightly slouched and empty-handed. In the central panel, the student had painted a loving Madonna, Mary the mother of Jesus, nestling her cheek against her infant boy. In the last panel stood an angel with a staff, who looked protectively over the other figures. Looking closely, one could see that these figures were composed of paper with printed text that had been torn into tiny pieces, applied to the wood, and then finally painted. In front of the triptych, the student placed a single votive candle.

The student was a nurse in our local hospital in its highly regarded NICU. While describing this work as often joyful and satisfying, she told the class about how she sometimes had to ask questions of mothers whose babies had died. She approached them with a clipboard in hand, filling out personal information about them and their now-dead child line by agonizing line. She recalled how she loathed this task, how invasive it felt, how she could not respond to their shock, pain, and sorrow. It was those same forms, now torn into small bits by her nurse's hands, which supplied the material of the triptych. "I never had the time to mourn for those mothers' losses, never had the time or space to feel their sadness. I had to get on with my job, including attending to other patients. Now I have a place to come to pray for those devastated mothers, to light a candle and offer them to God."

In her vulnerability and courage, this nurse taught me much about the unique burden healthcare professionals shoulder as they manage the many needs of patients or their families and bear witness to their suffering. She also underscored the need for all of us but particularly for medical staff to create spaces for mourning, to intentionally engage in the ancient practice of lament. In doing so, she refused to allow grief to determine the manner in which she performed necessary tasks. Her prayers also enabled her to connect to herself (e.g., acknowledging her frustration over bureaucratized health care, her awareness of the weight of a patient's or parent's loss, or her need to care during a shift for people in vastly different emotional and physical conditions). In this way, she could be sensitive to the sorrowful without diminishing the way she needed to also be present to other NICU families, such as those celebrating little lives that flourished against all odds. Accessing art and prayers from her Christian tradition, she practiced lament. In contrast to the nurse in our previous story, this student's heartache expanded compassion rather than contracted it, and intentional mourning freed her from grief's tyranny and its power to isolate.

Rather than stating that healthcare professionals best maintain professional distance, I am suggesting that their challenge is to attach to families in ways that befit caring in that particular moment. Of course, no one actually wants *mere* duty from those who deliver medicine; already vulnerable, we become more anxious when attended by the seemingly aloof doctor or the gruff nurse. But, clearly, we do not want staff to be so emotionally distraught over an infant's distress that they become paralyzed or ineffective. Rather than practicing either disassociation or emotional distancing, staff in these contexts should attach to their patient in the way that prioritizes their welfare and in ways befitting their unique role. The ability to do this requires what ethicists call "practical wisdom," that is, the learned capacity to do the right thing in the right way at the right time. For those working in the tender space of neonatal care, fostering this ability over the long term includes practicing lament and developing rituals that attend to grief's incessant knock on our heart's door.

Conclusion

When Susan spoke to one of my classes about their son and their journey with him, she noted, "It is tragic. But it is not *only* tragic." For Christians, God's loving, powerful presence with those who mourn keeps the pronouncement of their blessing from becoming twisted into the sick claim that loss itself is somehow salvific or therapeutic. The central symbol of our faith, a cross, has sometimes been misinterpreted in this way, as if it is an invitation to suffer for suffering's sake.[15] In the Mennonite tradition, the cross provides a way of naming tragedy honestly as well as a means of relativizing it. A rich image for Christians, the cross proclaims that there is much awry in the world, that humans sometimes heap evil upon one another, and that all creation—including tiny bodies whose chromosomes mysteriously misaligned—still yearns for healing. In this way, our story presses us to open ourselves to the weight of grief; that is, we can honestly call N.D.'s story a tragedy.

But as Susan noted, our story does not end in tears; nor does the cross forever bear the broken body of Christ. The cross also recalls for us the resurrection, pointing to "redemption," that is, to our conviction that God rescues us from what the psalmist descriptively dubs "the pit." (This assumes God sometimes does not keep us from falling into it; the psalms give us words to speak when we are trapped there.[16]) However odd it seems, Christians believe that God brings life out of death, that God eventually makes straight and true what was bent and broken. In particular, we believe that not even the deepest anguish can prevent the love of God from bringing forth good, particularly the good of union with one another in God.[17] Because we believe that this story is a truthful one, we invite our caregivers into it; thankfully, many medical staff willingly join with us as we seek to live as those open to the redemption of our tragedy. So, unlike the nurse who shut her eyes and ears to a mother's mourning, the hospital staff in Susan and Paul's case risked attaching to my friends. They entered into our story and witnessed the dedication that claimed a little dying boy as a beloved member of our community and also as someone destined for God's loving, re-storative embrace. By doing so, the medical team also claimed his broken body as their patient, as a boy worth the vulnerability that presence to dying infants necessitates.

Though it might seem counterintuitive, the biblical tradition of lament enacts profound hope by risking that God ultimately sustains us against the honest, utter force of our grief.[18] In this sense, Susan and Paul's son was indeed a gift not only to God but also to all of us—to his family, to our small Mennonite commu-nity, and to his medical team. He reminded us as people of faith of core, basic convictions often glibly proclaimed by us, convictions that we do not control our own lives, that to welcome children always entails exposing ourselves to pain, and that to love is to ultimately to know loss. N.D. reminded the NICU staff that attending to patients and families is always complex, an emotionally demanding task that invites providers to open themselves to the poignant beauty of these ever-so-fragile lives.

Noting that many of us wish to avoid displays of sorrow even at funerals, the poet and undertaker Thomas Lynch said, "Grief is the tax we pay on our attachments."[19] Healthcare providers attach by their presence to their patients or parents in exam rooms or the NICU; to honor the demands of grief, these providers can look for ways to provide space for rituals of lament for patients and families. But they must also create practices of mourning for themselves, acknowledging the vulnerability that dying, sick, or dead infants expose in all who seek to be fully alive. There is no magic formula, no "one size fits all" way for providers to foster sacred space for lament, and caregivers must mine their own resources, seeking counsel in their work contexts and from within their own faith traditions to care for patients and families —and themselves —wisely and well.

In closing, I offer the prayer composed on the occasion of the memorial celebration of N.D.'s short life (we were told not to wear black to his service by his parents). The prayer provides an example of how our evangelical, Anabaptist community sought to enact costly hope without dulling the sharp edge that cuts us all when we hold our anguish and open ourselves to the future—a future without an infant whom we held against our breast or whom we tended in our daily rounds.

Leader: What I feared has come upon me; what I dreaded has happened to me.
I have no peace, no quietness; I have no rest, but only turmoil.[20]
Congregation: *No peace, no quietness, no rest, but only turmoil.*
Leader: If only my anguish could be weighed and all my misery be placed on the scales!
It would surely outweigh the sand of the seas—no wonder my words have been impetuous.
Congregation: *Outweigh the sand of the seas.*
Leader: Yet if I speak, my pain is not relieved; and if I refrain, it does not go away.
Surely, O God, you have worn me out; you have devastated my entire household.
Congregation: *Devastated my entire household.*
Leader: To God belong wisdom and power; counsel and understanding are his.
Congregation: *Wisdom and power, counsel and understanding are his.*
Leader: At least there is hope for a tree:
if it is cut down, it will sprout again, and its new shoots will not fail.
Congregation: *It will sprout again.*
Leader: Its roots may grow old in the ground and its stump die in the soil,
yet at the scent of water it will bud and put forth shoots like a plant.
Congregation: *Put forth shoots like a plant.*
Leader: Oh, that my words were recorded, that they were written on a scroll,
that they were inscribed with an iron tool on lead, or engraved in rock forever!
I know that my Redeemer lives, and that in the end he will stand upon the earth.
Congregation: *I know that my Redeemer lives, and that in the end he will stand upon the earth.*
Prayer: Hidden God, in mystery and silence you are present in our lives, bringing new life out of death, hope out of despair. We thank you that you do not leave us alone but labor to make us whole. Help us to perceive your unseen hand in the

unfolding of our lives, and to attend to the gentle guidance of your Spirit, that we may know the joy of your love and rest in your peace. Amen.

Notes

1. Also called Patau syndrome, infants with this chromosomal abnormality suffer a number of severe physical and mental impairments such as heart disease and respiratory problems, and more than 90 percent of those who are born die within the first year. However, some Trisomy children live years. For reflections and photos of children and families who are living with this condition, visit http://trisomy.org.

2. Many Mennonites do not neatly fit into broader North American evangelicalism, especially because of the way it feels to us that evangelicalism too easily weds nationalism to Christian faith. Nonetheless, like a complicated family, Christian traditions overlap to create pockets of connection, such as our close relationship to those who also seek to trust in Christ, Scripture, and the Spirit in everyday life.

3. The phrase "in the shadow of the valley of death" is one translation of Psalm 23:4; the famous prayer begins, "The LORD is my shepherd, I shall not want."

4. The actual names of the couple have been changed, as have the names of all persons cited in this article.

5. For an accessible introduction to the Mennonite tradition, see http://thirdway.com/mennonites/who-are-the-mennonites/.

6. The *chesed*, lovingkindness, or steadfast love is among the most noted of God's characteristics in the Old Testament; see, e.g., Deut. 5:10, Nehemiah 9:30–33, or Psalm 86:5. Against the popular assertion that the Old Testament God is vindictive and vengeful, the overarching character of God belies this caricature. For an engaging, easy-to-read exploration of Israel's God, see, e.g., Ellen Davis, *Getting Involved with God: Rediscovering the Old Testament* (Cambridge, MA: Cowley, 2001).

7. By "orthodox" here, I mean core teachings of the church widely accepted over the ages and across cultures.

8. ". . . then the LORD God formed man from the dust of the ground and breathed into his nostrils the breath of life" (Gen. 2:7). Evangelicals need not interpret this literally to recall the truth that the breath of life is a gift—a miracle—that is also mysteriously withdrawn.

9. Orthodox Christianity affirms that God is not a man or a woman. Some of us occasionally utilize female pronouns to remind us of this truth.

10. Given that N.D. was born in respiratory distress, among other serious impairments, the willingness to allow him to die without medical interventions was relatively easy for this couple.

11. One hears this from Jesus on the cross, from which he cries out (quoting the first line of a lament psalm), "My God, my God, why have you abandoned me?" (Matt. 27:46). Jesus finds the experience of isolation amid his pain and humiliation most difficult to

bear, rather than the torture itself. The psalm from which he borrows his plea, Psalm 22, begins in this language of anguish, moves to proclaim God's eventual vindication of the afflicted, and ends with a hope of God's just reign over all. For Christians, Jesus models our assertion that Christian hope entails honest speaking of our lament, knowing that it takes place within God's larger, longer drama.

12. Matt. 5:4.

13. This is a simplistic explanation of Freud's insight about repression. Importantly, Freud acknowledged that we needed to sublimate some emotions or drives, most famously the sexual drive. But while sublimation channels and controls impulses so that we function well in society, repression sneaks up to sabotage our relationships with others and with ourselves. See, e.g., Freud's *Civilization and Its Discontents*. For ways this works in relationship to grief, see Elizabeth Kubler-Ross, *On Grief and Grieving: Finding Meaning through the Five Stages of Loss* (New York: Scribner, reprinted 2014).

14. This view might be more likely espoused by those who are not actually engaged in health care. Professionals know from experience that most of us do not live with emotions in compartments and recognize that "care" often entails some level of empathy; living this pragmatically and doing so wisely remain a challenge for all those in helping professions.

15. If one doubts this, see Matthew's Gospel in which Jesus pleads for an alternative to betrayal, torture, and the humiliating death on a cross (Matt. 26:37–46). Jesus models a love of life and does not seek out pain as an end in itself. Additionally, our Anabaptist tradition highlights that, by trusting in the resurrection rather than killing his enemies, Jesus vindicates all the innocent who long for justice amidst oppression or injustice.

16. One of the psalmists puts it this way, "The LORD . . . drew me up from the desolate pit, out of the miry bog, and set my feet upon a rock . . ." (Ps. 40:1–2).

17. Paul writes in one of his letters, "For I am convinced that neither death, nor life, nor angels, nor rulers, nor things present, nor things to come, nor powers, nor height, nor depth, nor anything else in all creation, will be able to separate us from the love of God in Christ Jesus our Lord" (Rom. 8:37–39).

18. There are many resources for lament. Within the Judeo-Christian tradition, Lamentations, as well as the Psalms, give voice to utter dejection, anguish, and loss. Leslie Allen weds his Old Testament scholarship to his many years as a hospital chaplain in his book, *A Liturgy of Grief: A Pastoral Commentary on Lamentations* (Grand Rapids, MI: Baker Academic, 2011).

19. In an interview with Bill Moyers years ago, Thomas Lynch commented that people commonly forbid the sending of flowers. In contrast, he was struck by the avalanche of bouquets at the death of Princess Diana, as if all the flowers we could not send in response to the death of our own loved ones found an outlet in response to her death. His point is that we want to avoid "taxes," and North American culture in particular fools itself into thinking we need not pay them without losing something more fundamental: our connection to one another. For links to documentaries of his life

and profession as well as his poetry and writing, see http://www.thomaslynch.com/1/234/index.asp.

20. The lament draws heavily from the book of Job, a notoriously difficult tale about terrible evils visited upon the innocent and the good—and really terrible theology and advice offered in the midst of them. In order of their allusion in the prayer, see Job 3:25–27; 6:2–3; 16:6–7; 12:13; 14:7–9; 19:23–25.

4

Spirituality in a Time of Crisis

A Protestant Christian Perspective

Ronald Cole-Turner

The birth of a high-risk infant often creates intense emotional stress for parents and their families. Facing such a situation, family members may find help and support by drawing on the resources of their religious or spiritual practices. The problem, however, is that the health crisis itself can undermine the basic assumptions upon which religious or spiritual support rests. It is even possible that the health crisis can become a spirituality crisis, exposing or increasing religious conflict between members of the family and undercutting the supportive benefits of spirituality. On the other hand, it is also entirely possible that the health crisis can be a moment of spiritual transformation and growth, one in which the parents or family members discover a more authentic and resilient spiritual awareness.

Spirituality, of course, is notoriously difficult to define, much less to manage. For most people, spirituality is interwoven into the complex fabric of life and therefore embedded in familial, communal, linguistic, and ritual systems, often in very complicated ways. In some form at least, religious belief or spiritual awareness is commonplace. But in today's environment of religious diversity, with multiple traditions and affiliations existing side by side, sometimes within the same family, it is impossible to speak of religion or spirituality in any simple or monochromatic terms. As hospital chaplains and medical practitioners know very well, many forms and degrees of religious conviction or spiritual practice can be present within one family.

All of this is complicated further by the fact that nurses and doctors bring their own spiritual or religious beliefs and experiences with them into the clinical setting. They should be encouraged to be self-aware about their personal attitudes and views about religion, positive or negative, particularly as they apply to the specific challenges posed by the birth of a high-risk infant. They should also be aware of the emotional and spiritual fatigue that can come upon them simply from doing their work well and should be encouraged to find ways to care for themselves in every dimension of their humanity.

After all, medical professionals cannot escape the fact that at least in minimal ways, they will be providing some form of spiritual care, whether they realize it or not. Simply by caring, simply by being fully present not just medically but *humanly*, in a manner that (one would hope) is warm and emotionally supportive, medical professionals offer care that has an implicitly spiritual dimension. By offering help with a human touch, good caregivers raise the spiritual and emotional warmth of a setting that might otherwise feel spiritually cold. Many caregivers will go so far as to recognize that "spiritual care is an essential component in providing support to NICU [neonatal intensive care unit] families."[1] According to at least one recent survey, "Most patients want their physicians or professional caregivers to address their spiritual and religious needs."[2] Whether implicit or explicit, religious convictions and spiritual awareness are never really absent from the complex caregiver–patient family dynamics of the clinical setting in which parents face the challenge presented by the birth of a high-risk infant.

The focus of this chapter, however, is not on spirituality in general or the complex forms it can take in a pluralistic culture but, rather, on some of the specific forms of spiritual life associated with the American Protestant religious experience. The objective is to increase the reader's awareness of how the challenge of the birth of a high-risk infant intersects with the assumptions and practices associated with "Protestant spirituality."

What Is "Protestant Spirituality"?

The idea that there is such a thing as "Protestant spirituality" is relatively new and not entirely familiar even to many Protestants. That is not to suggest that Protestant Christians have ever lacked for spiritual practices. From the early 1500s, these Christians have consistently emphasized the importance of a conscious and personal relationship with God maintained through activities such as reading the Bible or praying, either in groups or individually. Central to any notion of Protestant spirituality is a relationship with others and with God, often framed as a relationship with Jesus Christ, who is seen not just as a moral model or guide but as a confidant, an inner presence, and an intercessor. In these ways, Protestants look to Jesus Christ to mediate their spiritual relationship with God. If "spirituality" sounds like a new idea to Protestants, the need to develop a conscious awareness of a life-defining relationship with Jesus Christ is an old and much-valued idea.

While close to half of all Americans identify as Protestant Christians, it is important to note that there are divisions among various branches of Protestantism. For some Protestants, a spiritual connection with God is mediated through a sense of the presence and the power of the Holy Spirit. Often called Pentecostal and charismatic Christians, these believers are growing in numbers both inside and outside Europe and North America, and they are especially present among immigrant communities. Meanwhile, in the United States, African Americans are most often Protestant, usually Baptists or Pentecostals. Protestant churches in the United States remain largely segregated along racial lines. In terms of spirituality, African American Christians are more likely than their white counterparts to speak freely of their faith and of the sustaining role it plays in their lives and in the extended family and community. They are also more likely to speak of Jesus as a companion present in times of duress. At the same time, for reasons rooted in the history of racism in America, African Americans are sometimes wary of medical institutions or professionals, and this can intensify even more a strong reliance on religious communities in time of crisis.

It is important to note the varieties of Protestantism because this paper is focused mainly (but not exclusively by any means) on the historical forms of Protestantism that were organized in Western Europe and planted in North America in the colonial and federalist eras. Sometimes referred to as the "Protestant mainline," this includes traditional denominations such as Lutheran, Episcopalian, Presbyterian, Methodist, United Church of Christ (Congregational), and similar bodies. One thing these churches have in common is the practice of baptizing infants, a practice that bears directly on the central question of this paper. Most other Protestants believe that baptism is to follow a confession of faith and is therefore reserved for older children or adults.

The spiritual lives and practices of people today who identify with these traditional or "mainline" denominations are often understated or modestly expressed, as if too much religious talk or enthusiasm is best left to Christians of other persuasions. Despite this reticence or tendency to see religion as private, people today in these churches draw great strength from their communities, beliefs, and rituals.

The core challenge before us is that by whatever name and in whatever form this Protestant spirituality is known and practiced, it is the foundation of spirituality that is most challenged at a time of crisis and loss. "At times of crisis it is not surprising . . . that parents find their whole system of being in the world rocked and often shattered."[3] The health crisis presented by the birth of a high-risk infant challenges the very theology on which typical Protestant spirituality depends. It challenges the sense that we are connected to and being cared for by a loving God. In terms of personal emotional support, what is most needed is most threatened. To protect the theological foundation on which Protestant spiritual life is grounded, parents or family members are likely to respond to the crisis that follows the birth of a high-risk infant in any number of ways. The next section describes four such responses that are somewhat automatic or instinctive but are not especially helpful or sustainable over time.

Four Unsustainable Responses

When they first learn of the health crisis, Protestant parents are likely to find themselves asking how a loving and powerful God could let this happen. They will, of course, listen to the scientific and medical explanations. What are the biological processes that explain why their baby enters the world in such a tiny body or fragile state? Even if there is a straightforward biological explanation, it is not always easy to express it in clear and comprehensible terms. And even when the medical explanation is clear, space remains for unanswered questions that come more from the grieving heart than from a lack of medical information. For some parents more than others, this unfilled explanatory space cries out for other levels of explanation as it searches for hints of moral or spiritual meaning that can speak to the question, *Why?*

Some of the answers that come first to mind are not likely to be theologically strong or sustainable. They may help in a moment of crisis, but often one or more members of the family will sense that these initial responses are not based on the best parts of their core theological beliefs. For example, one of the first responses is to *blame oneself.* The mother or the father each might ask whether this is happening because of past behavior, perhaps from a past not fully disclosed. They may wonder: *Is my former failure coming due now, morally speaking? Is God punishing me or my spouse or the way we are together?*

Such morally causal thinking is perhaps not as common today as a century ago, but it is still present, in part because it contains a grain of truth. Bad choices often lead to pain and suffering. What is different here, however, is that the moral causality is divinely mediated. When someone drives too fast and strikes a pedestrian, the connection between the action and the pain and suffering that follow is obvious and undeniable. Imagine that someone generally drives recklessly, and God is said to want to teach her a lesson by sending a disease to someone in her family. That is a different kind of moral causality altogether because it requires divine mediation and depends on a theological view of a God who not only intervenes in nature but also specifically intervenes in order to punish us for our mistakes or sins.

Parents who respond by *blaming themselves* will likely come to a time of deeper reflection, whether in the moment or years afterward. Then, the thought that God is justified in harming the baby in order to punish the parent is turned into something else: God is blamed for being unfair. What starts as *blaming oneself* reduces to *blaming God*, which can be listed as the second of our four unsustainable explanations. Of the four, clearly this response is the most incompatible with spirituality. Who can trust in a God who has acted unfairly? It is a response so toxic to faith that almost no one will speak it aloud or entertain it long, unless of course it becomes the pivotal moment that triggers a life-changing rejection of faith.

A third unsustainable response is to *hope for a miracle*. The topic of miracles and divine intervention is something that divides Christians sharply, and these divisions can surface at a time of crisis. Christians know they should not see their faith as a kind of protection. They know there is no guarantee that being a good Christian means that divine protection is assured. But some Christians find it hard to dismiss that kind of thinking altogether. In many Christian communities, at least one person will be heard to say that those in need should look for a miracle, which they see as some sort of divine intervention that reverses the natural sequence of events and leads to a better ending.

Some Christians really do expect miracles, at least for those who show enough faith or who pray intensely. Stories of miracles circulate in some Christian communities, often with the commentary that miracles are forthcoming whenever the faith is strong and sincere. For some, a public display of strong faith can almost become a kind of spiritual bravado, put on in a moment of crisis in order to mask an inner lack of confidence or a deep fear of loss. If this happens, it can divide members of the family and create special challenges for the medical caregiver who feels a conflict between wanting to validate the beliefs of others and not wanting to give credence to wishful or delusional thinking. "It may be helpful [for clinicians] to begin a conversation with the family by validating their hope for a miracle. This is a way to acknowledge and respect another's beliefs, values, and faith. To do this genuinely, caregivers need to work through their internal resistance to miracle beliefs. One way of accomplishing this may be for caregivers to emphasize the search for common ground and acknowledge a shared commitment to the well-being of the baby."[4] It may also be helpful for caregivers to remember than even when extended family members or church friends may express publically their hope for a miracle, some of them may be silently wondering what a true miracle might actually look like under the circumstances.

A fourth unsustainable response is to see the entire crisis as *a test or trial* sent by God in order to help people grow. There is an obvious element of truth here in that the challenges of life do help people become more mature morally, psychologically, and spiritually. But many Christians who might entertain this idea for a time will reflect on it more deeply later, perhaps years later. Then they may come to reject the idea that *God sent this crisis for a purpose*. It is one thing for people to say that God helped them grow through this experience. It is quite another to think that God caused a health crisis for the newborn just to help the parents grow. Even so, some parents will be entertaining this idea as they live through this experience. But in the end, they may come to think that a God who teaches them at so heavy a cost is not worthy of worship.

These four responses—blame oneself, blame God, expect a miracle, or pass the test—are neither mutually exclusive nor sequential. Individuals and family members may find themselves in one frame of mind or another, perhaps stuck, perhaps moving quickly as the situation changes. They may reframe their interpretation or brace themselves in the face of mounting evidence or social pressure to modify their outlook. Members of the Christian clergy, whether or not they have a prior pastoral relationship with one or more family members, may endorse one or another of these four responses. The best clergy practice, of course, is to provide a constant and gentle presence that opens up the movement of parents through various unsustainable options to a more enduring and supportive spiritual awareness. One way this might be done is through the ancient Christian practice of baptism, described more fully in the next section.

Baptism in the Neonatal Intensive Care Unit

Among those Protestants today who accept and practice infant baptism, there is confusion and debate about what it actually means. From the start, Protestants rejected the sixteenth-century idea that unbaptized infants automatically go to hell if they die. For Protestants, infant baptism should have no urgency or existential anxiety attached to it. Its meaning lies in the way it welcomes the birth of the child within the community. In addition, infant baptism provides all members of the community with a dramatic and tangible reminder that divine grace, not human accomplishment, is the basis for hope of salvation.

Ordinarily, infant baptism occurs at a Sunday morning worship service with the congregation and the family in attendance, perhaps along with relatives or friends. As part of the worship, there is the "celebration" of infant baptism, a moment in which the baby's name is first given and spoken publicly in the context of worship. The scene is usually festive, the mood joyful, and the baby healthy. All this can be quite different when an infant baptism occurs in the NICU. The theological meaning and spiritual significance of a NICU baptism is also very different from the ordinary congregational experience, so much so that parents and family might wonder at first whether baptism is even appropriate under these unwanted circumstances.

What does infant baptism mean when it is "celebrated" in the life of the high-risk infant? Given the uncertain future of the infant, some will be tempted to reinstate the rejected view that baptism is a step necessary for salvation, something that must be done "just in case the baby dies." Classic Protestant theology denies this, but it is certainly held by many who call themselves Protestant. It is altogether likely that different people involved with the family will hold different views on this. But when infant baptism is de-linked from its medieval purpose of saving infants from hell, and yet occurs in the perplexing context of the NICU, it takes on an unexpected significance. Baptizing a high-risk infant signifies something different from the ordinary meaning associated with infant baptism. At first, a NICU baptism may seem confusing and out of place. It can, however, be a concrete action by the family and the family's faith community that claims that this human life, with all its uncertainties, is full of meaning.

Infant baptism ordinarily involves giving thanks for the gift of the child. It signifies the welcoming of the child into the community. In the context of the high-risk infant in the NICU, infant baptism requires some form of giving thanks to God for *this child with these limitations*. To acknowledge that this child is a gift goes against the obvious medical reality. The birth of the high-risk infant is in some respects the very opposite of what was anticipated. Birth and illness and perhaps even death come all at once. It is a birth without a future, at least not the future that was once envisioned and eagerly awaited by parents and grandparents as full of possibilities. What kind of a gift is this, so small, so fragile, so profoundly different from the gift first hoped for? This is a gift that appears to promise nothing but seems to demand everything.

To go against all appearances and to baptize *this child* is an act of witness to the reality of something more than meets the eye. It is an act of faith in the gift-like reality of the birth despite the obvious and painful truth of the reality that this gift is not at all the gift that was expected. It is to give a name to the child and, at the same time, to assign a meaning to the child's birth, to the child's condition, to the child's life no matter how brief or limited, and perhaps to the child's death. What meaning can there possibly be to such a life and such a death? Not the usual meaning, to be sure. This birth is not the start of something new and joyous and hopeful. It is the beginning and possibly the end at once, and for this very reason, because it compresses the entire human life span into a few days or weeks, baptizing such a life is an act of courage that reveals more than any ordinary baptism just what baptism signifies: an utter trust in God alone to provide the meaning of each individual human life.

And in that trust, parents who baptize such a child are declaring that *this* life—not the healthy version they imagined but this at-risk one they have been given—is now embraced and welcomed, held in their arms and enfolded into the as-yet-unwritten narrative of their lives, forever redefining them as the parents of *this* one. In naming this child, they are naming themselves as its parents. In that moment, they are consenting not to what they wanted but to what they have been given. This is now their life. When they participate in the baptism of their child, they are not trying to create meaning so much as trying to let themselves be overtaken by it.

Fragility and Spirituality

At our best, Christians agree that all our lives are fragile, vulnerable, and not very much in our control. The more we are aware of this, the more honest our theology and the more secure the foundation for a robust and resilient spirituality. In the awareness of weakness comes an awareness of strength from beyond the ordinary sources, a consciousness of the grace that comes most tangibly in moments of personal inadequacy. When they think about this, Christians often recall a little comment by the biblical writer Paul, who speaks of a time when he felt inadequate or too weak for his work. He writes that God reassured him with this word: "My grace is sufficient for you, for my power is made perfect in weakness."[5] Anyone who has experienced unexpected strength knows what this means. Christians sometimes interpret this awareness of inadequacy as *necessary* for the experience of grace.

There is another familiar text that is likely to come to mind during the health crisis of a high-risk infant. It is a story that begins with a disagreement between Jesus and his disciples about the importance of children:

> And they were bringing children to him, that he might touch them; and the disciples rebuked them. But when Jesus saw it he was indignant, and said to them, "Let the children come to me, do not hinder them; for to such belongs the kingdom of God. Truly, I say to you, whoever does not receive the kingdom of God like a child shall not enter it." And he took them in his arms and blessed them, laying his hands upon them.[6]

In a similar text, Jesus makes the stunning claim that, "Whoever welcomes one such child in my name welcomes me, and whoever welcomes me welcomes not me but the one who sent me."[7]

To picture Jesus as one who welcomes and blesses the little children is powerful enough on its own to provide assurance to some, but the point here goes even deeper. According to this text, Christians should see that we all need to become like little children. In what way? Perhaps by seeing a connection with a promise made by Jesus to be most clearly and fully present and identified with the weakest and most vulnerable members of the human community, or with "the least" among us, as the text puts it.[8] Another way to understand it is to connect it with Paul's comment about the grace that is experienced in weakness or vulnerability.

In the context of the birth of a high-risk infant, something extraordinary can occur. The weakness of the parents and their feelings of inadequacy can become a moment when they experience new strength. But more than that, something wholly unexpected and unexplainable can happen. The high-risk child, the one who is completely dependent on others, the one who in that moment is "the least of the least," becomes a grace-filled and transformative presence for others. For some parents, the fragility of the high-risk infant somehow becomes linked with Christ. Whether or not they recall Christ's promise to be present in the weakest or most needy, they find themselves being transformed by the little life entrusted to them.

Some parents may in time even see a connection between their fragile baby and the woundedness of Christ, and so they can come to see the one who is tiny and needy as a divine channel for an entirely unexpected encounter with spiritual healing. "The child is to be taken to the arms and welcomed, for the child is weak and needy. *The child thus represents Jesus as a humble, suffering figure.*"[9] These themes of Christian spirituality—Jesus' welcome to the children and advice that we should become like them, the presence of the divine in the most vulnerable, and our experience of God's strength in our own weakness—can flow together in unexpected ways in times of challenge and crisis.

Parents may find that they do not have the strength they need. And yet in that moment, in ways they probably cannot explain, they discover within themselves greater reserves of compassion and emotional strength than they ever knew existed. They find themselves facing demands they cannot meet and yet meeting them, finding capacities within themselves they did not know they had, perhaps in an unexpected ability to love in ways they could not have imagined even a few months before. In that moment, faced with demands they did not want and yet meeting them with strength of character they did not know they had, they find themselves alive perhaps as never before, awakened to their deeper or better selves and somehow inexplicably nourished in the challenge, however unwanted.

By being stretched, parents of high-risk newborns can find who they really are and what they are really made of. Or, perhaps more precisely, they can experience themselves being made into something more than they were. The fragile baby becomes unexpectedly Christ-like, changing others simply by being thrust upon them in such need.

A former NICU nurse who later became a seminary student reported just such an experience of inner spiritual transformation. In the course of her work as a nurse,

[s]he permitted herself to become attached to an infant born with trisomy 18, a serious chromosomal disorder that leads to death within a few months. . . . [She] wanted to take the infant, a girl whom she named Abby, into her home as a foster child. At first the state objected to a first-time foster mother taking a "special" child. Friends intervened, and Abby's brief life had the extraordinary effect of opening . . . [her] relationship with God so that "Abby" became,

as she recognized only later, her access to "Abba." Through her weakness, Abby transformed the one with power, the medical professional, by bringing her into a community of healing beyond power.[10]

It was years later that the nurse discovered that little Abby was in some wholly illogical way a tangible presentation of "Abba," which was the name Jesus used most often for God. It was not that the nurse's spirituality sustained her through this experience. Rather, the experience generated or evoked the spirituality. Without knowing why, she found herself named as the one to live for a time in the presence of this little, fragile one. Abby was "the least of the least," humanity in its most fragile state. For reasons that can only be described as grace, caring for the little one who was dying brought with it an awakening to a new dimension of life.

For parents and caregivers alike, human weakness and vulnerability in its tiniest form can awaken our deepest and best humanity. What is fragile becomes a pathway to something unexpected. Almost spontaneously, the little one in need cries out to be treated as precious and holy. When we respond to that cry, and when we create a sacred space for others to do so, we all become more profoundly human.

Notes

1. Joan L. Rosenbaum, Joan Renaud Smith, and Reverend Zollfrank, "Neonatal End-of-Life Spiritual Support Care," *Journal of Perinatal and Neonatal Nursing* 25, no. 1 (2011): 61–69, at 61.
2. Ibid., 61.
3. Ibid., 62.
4. Ibid., 65.
5. 2 Corinthians 12:9; RSV.
6. Mark 10:13–16.
7. Ibid., 9:37.
8. See Matthew 25.
9. Judith M. Gundry-Volf, "The Least and the Greatest: Children in the New Testament," in *The Child in Christian Thought*, ed. Marcia J. Bunge (Grand Rapids, MI: William B. Eerdmans, 2001), 29–60, at 44–45.
10. Ronald Cole-Turner and Brent Waters, *Pastoral Genetics: Theology and Care at the Beginning of Life* (Cleveland, OH: Pilgrim, 1996), 153, n. 17.

5

Muslim Biomedical Ethics of Neonatal Care

Theory, Praxis, and Authority

Zahra Ayubi

Long before anti-Muslim sentiment heightened in the United States with the 2016 presidential election, Muslim patients and their families worried that healthcare professionals might compromise their care if they harbored anti-Muslim sentiment, which prevails in American political and social discourses.[1] The current political climate accentuates the ethical imperative to bioethicists and medical personnel to learn about Muslim beliefs and practices in order to provide care that is not only the best medically but is also culturally sensitive. In this chapter, I discuss the Muslim biomedical ethics of what is arguably among the most precarious of medical situations: neonatal care for cases in which infant demise is imminent.

The diagnosis of a fetus or baby with serious developmental defects or fatal abnormalities, where survival is or will be limited to a number of days or even hours and minutes, poses difficult Islamic ethics questions to Muslim parents and their medical teams.[2] These questions may include: should the pregnancy be allowed to continue? if the infant is allowed to come to term, what are the Islamic birth and death rites? and when is it ethically permissible to withdraw intensive neonatal care? These questions have arisen as a result of advances in fetal screening technologies and intensive neonatal care that are making the age of viability, the ability to survive outside the womb, earlier. Attempts at formulating answers to these questions are important both for helping caregivers and Muslim parents determine an Islamic, ethical course of action and for contributing perspectives from neonatal care to the broader corpus of the still inchoate field of Islamic biomedical ethics.

Yet, questions of what should happen in terms of birth and death rites, mourning, and even withdrawal of medical care for infants with definitely limited futures are relatively uncomplicated from an Islamic ethicolegal standpoint; rather, the course of action that should be taken is complicated by differing Muslim practices, which serve as competing discourses. What Muslims may believe in textually may be distinct from Muslim praxis, and biomedical ethics decisions may be based upon either texts or practices that Muslims have observed. A chosen course of action also hinges on who is making the decisions. In this chapter, I argue that bioethicists and medical practitioners should be aware of differences between ethicolegal theory and ethical praxis in decision making in neonatal care—that it is important to be familiar with theoretical Islamic biomedical ethics but to be aware that Muslim beliefs and practices cannot be reduced to the teachings of texts.[3]

Muslim beliefs and practices are diverse. Because the global Muslim community of 1.6 billion[4] subsumes multiple regions, cultures, sects, and levels of observance, there is no singular description of Muslim birth and death rites. The American Muslim community is also arguably a microcosm of this global Muslim diversity, in that Muslims from all over the world have been living in the United States for generations, sometimes intermarrying with other Muslims and non-Muslims, too—resulting in various practices as well as gender norms that are all at play in the care of Muslim patient families in the United States.

Still, I have developed two parallel but related ethical models that demonstrate how Muslim families of various cultural backgrounds, sects, or religiosity might incorporate their religious traditions into neonatal medical decisions. The first, which I call the Scriptural-Dependent model, is based on ethicolegal theory as exposited in texts. The second is the Ritual-Dependent model, which is based on Islamic birth and death rituals. I outline the Scriptural-Dependent model by describing the main juristic and religioethical positions that bioethicists and many doctors and patient families draw on regarding the status, rituals, and treatment of newborns with fatal abnormalities or short survival time. Following this, I describe the Ritual-Dependent model through findings from empirical biomedical ethics studies on Muslim families' decision making for neonatal care of such infants. This handful of cross-cultural studies in Muslim communities worldwide is specifically designed to demonstrate to medical staff that Western biomedical ethics guidelines do not work when counseling Muslim families and to propose alternative guidelines based on clinical experience with Muslim families. Though few in number, the empirical studies are also telling of the gender dynamics that can overrun decision making about what should happen in cases of unavoidable death of a neonate.

After discussing the two models of Muslim beliefs and praxis, I provide practical advice to staff about questions related to the elements involved in the ethics of neonatal care for Muslim families—namely, care and care-withdrawal options, questions about religious authority figures and decision making, and follow-up upon bereavement. Which model a patient's family may lean toward for care, death rites, and bereavement, or perhaps a combination of the two models or another perspective entirely, is largely a question of who holds religious authority in the eyes of the family and what elements, if any, of the Islamic tradition they deem relevant. Religious authority, decision-making power in cases of neonates with fatal abnormalities, and death rites and bereavement are bound up with gender dynamics and male normativity.

The empirical studies also reveal, but do not always specifically comment on, many clinicians' observation that fathers or other male family members tend to make unilateral decisions, often but not always in consultation with doctors and sometimes imams (religious leaders) or Muslim scholars ('alims). Male family members may consult Muslim religious authority figures on issues such as what care a neonate should receive, what care should be withheld or withdrawn, and what birth and death rites are to be performed, if any—sometimes to the complete exclusion of and psychological harm to the grieving, postpartum mother. Some of the studies, particularly ones authored by the medical anthropologist Alison Shaw, which I discuss later, reveal great familial pressure on mothers that comes in the form of Islamic biomedical counsel during various stages of decision making. Given empirical evidence that once a fetus leaves a woman's body, patriarchal cultural expectations and gendered power differentials dominate discourse surrounding care of severely developmentally challenged neonatal infants, I argue that practitioners' recognition of maternal decision-making power is critical in order to have an egalitarian biomedical ethics.

Personhood in the Scriptural-Dependent Model

The options for care, care withdrawal, and death rites all hinge on the point at which a fetus is considered a person. The paradigm of care that I call the Scriptural-Dependent model is centered on understandings of personhood that emerge from verses of the Qur'an (Muslim scripture) or *hadiths* (posthumously recorded sayings by the Prophet Muhammad). Islamic bioethics uses the term *ensoulment* to refer to the moment when God breathes *ruh* or spirit into a fetus.[5] This is referred to in Qur'anic verses and *hadiths* about the stages of fetal development as signs of God's mercy. Qur'an verses 23:12–14, which outline stages of human creation that are parallel to fetal development, translate to:

> Verily, We created the human from an essence of clay; then placed him as a seed-drop firm in a resting place; then We fashioned the seed-drop into a clot, then We fashioned the clot into an embryonic lump, then We fashioned the embryonic lump into bones, then clothed the bones with flesh, and then it is produced as another creation. So blessed be Allah, the Best of creators.

Qur'an 32:7–9, still referring to developmental stages, mentions a moment in which God breathes spirit into a fetus:

> The One Who made all things good He created good, He began the creation of man from clay. Then He made his offspring from an extract of insignificant water. Then He fashioned him and breathed into him of His Spirit; and appointed for you the hearing and the sight and the feelings. What little thanks you give.

In a *hadith* that is largely read by bioethicists as superimposing a timeline onto this fetal development, Prophet Muhammad specifies that forty days elapse between each of these stages, so that 120 days elapse before the Qur'anic references to a being "produced as another creation" and the breathing in of God's spirit. The *hadith* reads:

> Each one of you is constituted in the womb of the mother for forty days, and then he becomes a clot of thick blood for a similar period, and then a piece of flesh for a similar period. Then Allah sends an angel who is ordered to write four things. He is ordered to write down his deeds, his livelihood, his (date of) death, and whether he will be blessed or wretched (in religion). Then the soul is breathed into him. . . .[6]

Based on these scriptural sources, most legal schools of thought state that ensoulment occurs 120 days after conception, which also happens to be approximately the time when a mother begins to feel fetal movement, or quickening. As Vardit Rispler-Chaim explains, it is also at this 120-day point that jurists consider the fetus a legal person who can inherit, leave an inheritance to its relatives if it dies in utero, or permit the mother to receive blood money if someone causes maternal injury resulting in fetal death.[7] In other words, the fetus is considered a legal person after 120 days of gestation.

Theoretically, the medical care options for infants with fatal abnormalities resemble those of any patient facing imminent death, especially since such an infant is older than 120 days from the point of conception. In other words, a severely compromised neonate's life is legally the same as anyone else's life. The salient religioethics question is: to what kind of care should a neonate's family consent if they know that death is imminent? To this question, a different set of Qur'anic verses is relevant. Namely, verse 5:32, which bioethicists have referred to in end-of-life care discourses, states, "Whosoever has taken a human life, it is as if he has taken the life of humankind." Some empirical studies have shown that considering this verse and the Islamic jurisprudential principle of preserving life, some Muslim families categorically reject ever withdrawing care.[8]

In addition to this verse, the verse prohibiting female infanticide (81:8–9) and verses prohibiting killing one's children for financial survival (6:151 and 17:31) may be cited in cases of infant patients. But the discourse on neonates differs from many end-of-life discourses in that death is naturally imminent, regardless of treatment or its withdrawal, which may not be the case for all adults. In cases of imminent death for adults, when treatment is futile, most jurists permit its withdrawal.[9]

In contrast, the imminence of death has led some neonatal intensive care unit (NICU) clinicians in Muslim countries to develop guiding principles that are rooted in the scriptural model for counseling families. They recommend that medical staff emphasize the ideas that: (1) letting the natural course of action take place is not the same as withdrawing care or killing the child because (2) the reality of the fatal abnormalities is that treatment, surgical or otherwise, does not make a difference. Further, (3) modern medicine and physicians' abilities, they emphasize, are limited and cannot control what is inevitable, or decreed by God, referring to the *hadith* of the pre-decreed moment of death.[10] The studies also recommend that nutrition, pain medication, and even ventilation be maintained (in cases in which use of the ventilator does not affect outcomes) so that death comes naturally, without extraordinary intervention. Costa, Ghazal, and Al Khusaiby, cited previously, feel that the very act of discussing the significance of do not resuscitate (DNR) orders in light of observing an inevitable outcome pre-decreed by God, regardless of the intervention, is the way for clinicians to handle biomedical ethics questions that Muslim families may have that is most proximate to Islamic biomedical ethics principles. However, while these guidelines draw on scriptural references, quoting them may or may not be welcome. The likelihood of parents' considering these ideas, particularly when articulated by non-Muslim clinicians, might be increased if they are cited in a framework of a shared desire to "figure out" a decision together that is culturally sensitive. On the other hand, a patient's family may question the motives of clinicians who make heavy-handed references or claims to knowledge of the Islamic way in order to advocate the withdrawal of care.

Post-mortem care, burial rites, or bereavement are not always topics in Islamic medical ethics that *fatwa* literature (legal responsa by scholars of Islamic jurisprudence) addresses because they are mostly concerned with what to do for the living. *Fatwas*, both historical and recent ones on after-death care, vary slightly on details. For the most part, they agree that any baby, whether miscarried, stillborn, or born alive, who dies after the 120 days of gestation, when ensoulment occurs, should be given a name; have a *janaza*, or Muslim funerary prayer, performed at a mosque or cemetery in front of the body; and be buried as promptly as possible. Jurists disagree over whether the body must be washed before shrouding and burial. Some hold that because infants are considered sinless and therefore pure, their bodies need not be washed, while others hold that they must be washed to purify themselves from coming into contact with the mother's blood (an impure substance).[11] Typical Muslim customs require prompt burial because of respect for the body, which belongs to God and which must be returned to God as soon as possible after physical demise—usually within 24 to 48 hours. Generally, Muslim jurists have permitted autopsies if the cause of death is unknown or if there is knowledge to be gained that will prevent future deaths.[12] Muslim burials are typically "green burials," meaning the body is shrouded in a cloth of natural fibers, usually by family members of the same sex (though the sex of those who prepare the body does not matter in the case of infants), and committed to the ground according to local custom, without a coffin. If local laws do not permit "green burials," Muslims typically make use of the thinnest wooden coffin allowed by local burial codes. After burial, there is typically a mourning period[13] and a variety of bereavement practices, which vary widely according to local cultures, such as a show of community support through visits to the grieving parents' home, delivery of meals to the family, and in-home, mosque-based, or gravesite recitations of the Qur'an by friends and family.[14]

Ritual-Dependent Model

The Ritual-Dependent model of care options and death rites is also concerned with the point at which a baby is considered a person but defines personhood as the ability to receive birth rites. This definition-cum-understanding of person-hood, in turn, carries much more complex implications for care decisions and bereavement because one has to make judgment calls about the fetus's ability to receive birth rites as well as about who carries the authority to make such calls.

Many birth and death rites across various Muslim traditions originate in the *sunnah* (practices of the Prophet Muhammad) and *hadith* that diversely manifest in cross-cultural and sectarian practices of Muslim communities. While practices vary, there are two universal ones that occur immediately at birth: naming the baby and recitation of the call to prayer (*adhan*) in the ears of the baby. In most Muslim families, the father of the infant or other patriarch of the family (such as a maternal or paternal grandfather) recites the call to prayer, although a mother or matriarch may do so in some instances. Typically, most Muslim families across all cultures practice male circumcision, though depending on the community, it does not always take place immediately following birth.[15] In the United States, many Muslim families commonly choose to have circumcisions done at the hospital before the baby is discharged. In addition, typically, within six days of birth, or at any point in childhood, financially able parents donate the meat of one or two sheep or other livestock to charity; this is often, though not in all Muslim cultures, accompanied by a celebration of the birth at home and shaving of the hair that the baby is born with. If an infant dies, as I mentioned previously, there should be a prompt burial, in which a minimal coffin is preferred in most cases.

In the Ritual-Dependent model, care withdrawal might depend on whether drawing an independent breath is the standard for establishing personhood. If the fetus is not expected to live long enough to receive the call to prayer, or if abnormalities preclude the ability to breathe or hear, even if there is a prolonged period before the official time of death, then the infant's personhood might not be established in the family's perspective. Therefore, these families may not feel that withholding care is tantamount to taking a life. That is, if personhood is not established for a given family because of the infant's inability to receive the call to prayer, the family may choose to withhold care altogether or partially. This was the case for a father in Alison Shaw's study who requested doctors to "just keep the tubes and medicines, but . . . no ventilator . . . it's up to her, we will see if she has the will to live . . . and . . . I could see . . . it was too much for her."[16] Because the neonate did not draw an independent breath and hear the call to prayer, the family did not interpret her as being a "person" and thus also forwent formal funeral rites. However, for some, live birth may blur that line of establishing personhood, and they may choose to provide life-sustaining care, even if they believe that lack of receiving the call to prayer or a short life span determined nonpersonhood for them.

The most notable differences in the scriptural- and ritual-based models of determining personhood are the funerary and bereavement processes. Allison Shaw's study shows that at least in some Muslim cultures, there is some confusion on the part of parents as to what procedure to follow for miscarried babies, stillborn babies, and live births, which speaks to the heart of when some Muslims define full personhood, independent of the notion of 120 days.

Defining the moment of personhood matters for one's understanding of the nature and gravity of loss. In an article that argues that the "right not to be born" should be included in biomedical ethics discourse, Vardit Rispler-Chaim states that, "when there is no 'personhood' no rights [as in legal rights] are due."[17] Shaw, who conducted a study on experiences with infant death among Kashmiri-Pakistani women in the United Kingdom, found that her interlocutors associated the beginning of new life with the experience of feeling fetal movement, consistent with Qur'anic and legal interpretation in the scriptural model, but that their families and communities only considered live birth as a marker of full personhood because of the possibility of speaking the call to prayer into the baby's ear.[18] Shaw found that this difference in definitions of personhood affected medical decisions because of the chance to have publically acknowledged grief.

Shaw describes an interlocutor, Sameena, whose first baby died after three days and was given a full *janaza* (funeral prayer and burial rites) and whose second baby died in utero at forty weeks (full term). Even though in Islamic law and in Islamic biomedical ethics literature, life beyond 120 days marks the baby as a "person," her family did not observe any funeral rites for that second baby, possibly because they were unaware of the 120-day benchmark or because they considered the rituals associated with establishing personhood as more important. In Sameena's third pregnancy, her fetus was again diagnosed with fatal abnormalities. In light of her prior experiences, she decided both to continue with the pregnancy and to have an early cesarean delivery so that the baby could draw breath and thus be considered by her family as a whole person, deserving of funeral rites. So the notion of personhood and corresponding burial rites affected the mother's medical decisions, namely of whether to continue an ill-fated pregnancy and when to schedule a cesarean delivery (or, in other cases, when to induce labor). Unfortunately, her physicians dismissed her desire to deliver early as religious and not medically necessary, and the baby, like her second, was also stillborn close to term. She laments: "My husband and parents would not recognize him as a person to be named because he had not drawn breath. So I named him myself. He is buried in the snowdrop garden," a cemetery for stillborn infants.[19] She continues, "If he had drawn even one breath, then we would have had a funeral, all the family would have been there . . . but no, it's like he never existed," and thus, neither did her grief. Because drawing breath and receiving the call to prayer are essential to establishing personhood in the ritual-based model of Muslim practice, the lack of funerals and communally recognized period of bereavement carries long-lasting psychological effects on mothers and potentially others in the family. Which model a family follows might be culturally determined or dependent on the dominant positions that religious authorities they trust take.

Maternal Rights, Bereavement, and Religious Authority

Regardless of the kinds of authority involved, they are deeply bound up with historical notions that paternal power supersedes maternal power. Religious historian Kathryn Kueny argues that historically in Muslim societies, reproduction, attending births, and all things relating to maternity have been the provenance of midwives, grandmothers, and other maternal figures. She shows, however, that male scholars'

assert[tion] of control over the maternal body suggests a certain level of discomfort with the Qur'anic ideal that God creates in wombs whatever, and however, he pleases, . . . In order to privilege their own procreative power, men usurp God's omniscience and omnipotence through a variety of authoritative discourses to guarantee the entire reproductive process is directed toward their desired outcome. . . .[20]

Historically, male scholars have used religious discourses to reassert male authority over reproduction in rejection of the previously held exclusivity of women caring for women in childbirth. Aside from these premodern scholarly attempts at control, in many Muslim societies, female control over maternity ended with colonialism and the medicalization of reproduction that placed the field of gynecology in the hands of men (Western only at first) and male decision makers (even if individual doctors are now women).[21]

Empirical studies show that mothers are also frequently denied being fully informed of the medical condition of their baby and treatment and withdrawal of treatment options from Islamic bioethics perspectives. A study from Oman designed to aid medical practitioners to develop sensitivity in working with Muslim families on instituting DNR orders or a care withdrawal plan for their neonate states that their counseling sessions were conducted either with "both parents or [the] father alone."[22] In addition to instituting DNR orders, the Oman study also recommends that an "elderly male who may be a close relative or a cleric" should be present, suggesting that, ultimately, the right conclusions can be reached if male authority figures guide them.[23] One of Shaw's male interlocutors, Talib, whom I discussed earlier as someone who followed the Ritual-Dependent model, did so in consultation with a *pir* (a religious elder, or one's personal religious teacher), whom he had invited to visit the baby in the NICU to help him decide whether to discontinue life support. As I recalled earlier, based on his recommendation, the father instructed the doctors to take the infant off the ventilator but continue medications to see whether she would live.[24] Shortly after, "he simply told his family, including his wife that 'the baby died.'"[25] The mother was not informed of any treatment measures or decisions until after her child's death and thus had no part in the Islamic biomedical ethics discussion that did take place, but only between father and *pir*. This calls into question how ethical the decision could have been.

It is possible that in certain family situations, such as Talib's and those in the Omani study, the mothers were indisposed, were undergoing their own health complications, or wished not to be included in the decision making out of grief. However, this logic of "shielding" women from decision making is a paternalistic apologetic for denying them autonomy or religious authority. Contrary to this thinking, a study by Anita Lundqvist and Anna-Karin Dykes quotes their participants, Muslim mothers, as saying about being informed, "It is good to be informed concerning how the baby will be treated, drugs etc. The mother needs to know." and "Yes, I have to be informed why they will withdraw. . . . How difficult it is for the baby. What is happening, why they do not want to go on . . . and how it will be performed."[26] Another said, "Yes, if it is of use for the baby, one has to accept [to take part in care]. I will not think of myself as breast-feeding if the baby needs tube feeding. I will do it. All I can do as a mother for the baby I will accept."[27] Finally, one stated, "I want[ed] to be there with my baby, but it was very trying for me. . . ."[28] In other words, with information, mothers are able to participate in the care and care withdrawal processes and assert their agency in deciding how much to be involved, all of which later affects the conditions of their bereavement. A female gynecologist in the United Kingdom, Fatima Husain, wrote a paper reporting her success in guiding vulnerable Muslim women through nonaggressive neonatal management because they were able to use their autonomy in decision making.[29] She states,

> In all these cases, the obstetric, midwifery and neonatal staff provided individualized care with continuity at consultant level for the important decisions regarding fetal assessment, monitoring, mode of delivery and resuscitation. The whole team caring for these very vulnerable women could therefore help them through a traumatic experience. No assumptions were made about which route the women would follow despite awareness of their cultural and religious backgrounds; these women, supported by their families, would have to live with the consequences of their decisions.

The lack of assumptions on the part of Husain's medical team and of respect for the decision-making autonomy of the women is for Husain the element that provides "ethical dimensions" to cases of fatal abnormalities in infants.

Indeed, along with informed consent, the availability of religious ethics discourses may prevent some families from coming to the juncture of having to decide on care options for severely compromised neonates—that is, they may choose abortion upon learning of fatal abnormalities. The empirical studies on Muslim families show that despite the existence for at least three decades of *fatwas* permitting abortion past 120 days in such cases, both Muslim practice and counsel from medical staff and Muslim imams and elders dissuade women from opting for abortion. Alison Shaw explains that at least in the United Kingdom, "medical practitioners think there is no point in offering prenatal diagnosis to Muslim patients because [they think] Islam unconditionally forbids termination of pregnancy."[30] Shaw's interlocutors also showed lack of knowledge on the subject. A woman named Shakeela "sought unsuccessfully to find any authoritative Islamic support to enable her to end a first pregnancy shown on ultrasound to have multiple fatal abnormalities [fluid in the lungs and brain, and abnormalities of the heart]."[31]

She explains in her interview,

> I thought I might [have the abortion . . .], but my Mum said in our religion termination is a sin, it is murder and God will punish you after death, unless it is certain the mother will die . . . otherwise it is not allowed. My mum said she would look after the baby if it is handicapped. . . . My Dad told me to pray. He said, "the doctors aren't always right. . . ."[32]

Books she found in her parents' home confirmed that abortion is only allowed in case of mortal danger to the mother. She then contacted a relative who was married to an al-Azhar University–trained imam who refused to discuss the matter with her, even though that couple had terminated their third pregnancy upon detection of fatal abnormalities. Shaw concludes that because Shakeela did not find "Islamic support for [terminating], she did not end this pregnancy."[33] The birth was a traumatic experience for Shakeela, particularly because of the baby's appearance. Shaw writes,

> with her pyramid-shaped head, 2.5 litres of liquid having been removed from her brain, and a rib emerging from her belly . . . both parents and the birth attendants were frightened, so much so that the mother regretfully recalled that "I did not even kiss her." The baby was named, lived for less than an hour and subsequently was buried in the Muslim cemetery.[34]

At the funeral, Shakeela learned from relatives who suffered similar trauma about legal opinions permitting abortion in such cases and commented, "it's a shame people don't discuss these things. Why don't they discuss it on digital or on TV? Or even have some leaflets about Islam and abortion. So many people don't know what to do. They say Islam has a solution for everything, so why are there no guidelines for this?"[35] Clearly, Shaw's interlocutor Shakeela is concerned about pregnant women's access to Islamic biomedical ethics literature, without which someone like her would allow family, community, or elders to decide for them. Several others of Shaw's interviewees, as well as Muslim women survey-takers in another empirical study on neonatal end-of-life care from Sweden by Lundqvist and Dykes, described their family's pressure to maintain a pregnancy in cases of diagnosis with fatal abnormalities. In the view of those families, Islam does not allow for abortion, and women should as mothers simply accept fate as God decreed.[36] So, it is not just that there is a gap in theoretical discussion of abortion ethics and Muslim practice, but women would *like to be informed* about the full range of options according to Islamic legal thought.

Most religious scholars across various sects are unanimous about the permissibility of abortion in cases of danger to the mother's life. Many, based on Qur'anic verses and *hadith,* say that a breastfeeding woman may terminate a subsequent pregnancy because it is believed that the "living child has priority [of receiving nutrition] over the fetus," though this permission is not universal and, again, must take place before 120 days—reiterating that a fetus is considered a living child only after the 120-day mark.[37] More relevant: since the 1980s, muftis from several countries, including Kuwait, Saudi Arabia, Iran, and Pakistan, have ruled that abortion is permissible if fatal abnormalities, genetic disorders leading to a severely compromised life, or severe physical or mental defects are detected—some argue before three months, some maintain the 120-day mark, and some even have ruled permissibility after 120 days.[38] Several muftis emphasize that this latter dispensation is for serious defects, not handicaps that would allow a relatively normal life such as blindness or absence of a hand.[39] A few scholars hold that genetic diseases or incurable diseases are not grounds for abortion because a cure may be found in the child's lifetime.[40] To sum up, as it pertains to cases of neonatal care for infants with limited futures, the discussion about abortion helps us to establish notions of when personhood begins in biomedical jurisprudence and clarify that there is a body of literature that would have permitted abortion in such cases.

However, I need to make clear that I am not arguing for the standard forms of religious authority to be upheld—it is not that if imams just studied up on biomedical ethics questions, and if Muslims just followed "traditionally" produced knowledge, everything would be fine. Rather, I am arguing that mothers' experience and motherhood itself ought to be considered valid forms of authority. It is not that if Muslims just followed the law, then Islamic ethical decision-making would be made possible. Women's desire to discuss religioethical issues openly signals their desire to assess religious ethics itself, to discuss their experiences within it, and to talk about their particular circumstances in order to have an ethics that speaks to their situation.

For a clinician, any power asymmetry between the mother and father, and even a religious cleric, may not be an important issue. However, if the empirical evidence I cited earlier serves as a series of cautionary tales, there is an ethical imperative for clinicians to include women in decision making in order to make any potential application of religious ethics also gender egalitarian, which I argue will make decisions more ethical. This can be done by ensuring that both parents (or those who would be the legal guardians of the child) are present for all medical updates given by staff, that both are given complete information about treatment and care options, that both are present for any ethics discussions and consultations with religious authorities, and that both consent to decisions, even if the presence and consent of only one parent are required by law or hospital policy. Updating NICU protocols to reflect gender parity in informing parents and requiring joint decisions can be invaluable in making sure that the insistence to speak to both parents does not come off as paternalistic insistence. Rather, it can be a matter of policy, if not legally according to hospital regulations, then part of the NICU culture. It is not unprecedented in Muslim countries for hospitals to encourage greater gender parity as a policy so that patient families may make more egalitarian, and therefore ethical, decisions.[41] Additionally, female staff members can play the subtle role of making sure Muslim mothers feel informed about their neonates' status and are contributing to any bioethics decisions, being aware of, but *not assuming*, potential power differentials between Muslim mothers and fathers.

Clinicians cannot assume that religious clerics, such as local imams, might be able to help patient families make decisions, perhaps because they may lack the training or may not be welcome in such sensitive episodes in a family's life, or they may be of a different sect. Even when consulted, religious clerics may defer to medical professionals, as we saw in some of the empirical studies, because they may be uncomfortable with making decisions on uncommon scenarios about which they may not have had the opportunity to formulate opinions or have access to jurisprudential literature on the subject. They may just provide comfort and perform funerary rites. Nonetheless, forging relationships with local Muslim scholars, imams, or community elders on the premises that they must be willing to speak to both parents, as well as asking about forming partnerships with female scholars or other active female members of the local Muslim community, is an important first step in identifying religious authorities who could be gender conscious.

Conclusion

The key to understanding Muslim biomedical ethics of neonatal care is to recognize that there is great diversity of thought and practice. Muslims are not their scripture. That is, they may or may not follow scripture or law, even if they are religious. The sorrow of having an infant with fatal abnormalities may suspend ideas of what decisions they "should" make according to religious beliefs or who should be consulted. Many Muslim families may make decisions on their own in fear that religious authorities might be too conservative and may not permit the withdrawal of care that doctors may be recommending. Or perhaps they may not want the attention, or they may not want their community to become aware of their situation. On the other hand, they may want community support to help them grieve.

There are, however, ethical considerations in decision making on care and care withdrawal in the NICU. Clinicians should show familiarity with Islamic bio-medical ethics concerns (not answers or rulings) that might be at play in Muslim families' decision-making processes. For families that do want consultation with religious authorities to decide on care withdrawal, and do come to a decision to withdraw care, it will likely be comforting to speak of the Islamic bioethics principle drawn from the *hadith* that each person's moment of death is already decreed, regardless of interventions.

As some scholars of Islamic bioethics have found to be the case in Muslim countries, families may in fact ask clinicians if they know anything about Islamic bioethics to help them with decision making, or provide references to someone they may consult.[42] Best practices would be to provide families with literature on Islamic biomedical ethics from a variety of perspectives, offer contacts not just to religious clerics such as local imams but also potentially to Islamic bioethicists, and make sure that both parents, including the mother, are fully informed of the infant's condition and the ethical questions that may emerge for the families. Empirical evidence shows that women need to be fully informed for the sake of maternal respect as well as for their bereavement process. Care providers, religious authorities, and families can all make Muslim experiences in the NICU more ethical.

Notes

1. Muslim families in other non-Muslim majority countries may feel this as well.
2. A few examples of such infants are those who manifest Trisomy 13 or 18, or Lesch-Nyhan syndrome, all for whom death in infancy is a certainty.
3. Reducing Muslim beliefs and practices to one particular reading of selective Islamic texts was a hallmark of Orientalist thought of the eighteenth through early twenty-first centuries.
4. As of 2010, the global Muslim population is estimated at 1.6 billion. That number is thought to have grown to 1.8 billion now. See http://www.pewresearch.org/fact-tank/2017/01/31/worlds-muslim-population-more-widespread-than-you-might-think/.
5. Abdulaziz Sachedina, *Islamic Biomedical Ethics: Principles and Application* (Oxford: Oxford University Press, 2009), 102, 139–41.
6. Sahih al-Bukhari no: 3036.
7. Vardit Rispler-Chaim, *Islamic Medical Ethics in the Twentieth Century* (Leiden: E. J. Brill, 1993), 9.
8. Anna E. Westra, Dick L. Willems, and Bert J. Smit, "Communicating with Muslim Parents: 'The Four Principles' Are Not as Culturally Neutral as Suggested," *European*

Journal of Pediatrics 168, no. 11 (November 2009): 1385. This study effectively shows that the widely accepted Four Principles of biomedical ethics of autonomy, nonmaleficence, beneficence, and justice cannot be universally imposed.

9. Sachedina, 170.

10. A. R. Gatrad, B. J. Muhammad, and A. Sheikh, "Reorientation of Care in the NICU: A Muslim Perspective," *Seminars in Fetal and Neonatal Medicine* 13, no. 5 (October 2008): 312–14; D. E. Da Costa, H. Ghazal, and Saleh Al Khusaiby, "Do Not Resuscitate Orders and Ethical Decisions in a Neonatal Intensive Care Unit in a Muslim Community," *Archives of Disease in Childhood—Fetal and Neonatal Edition* 86, no. 2 (2002): 115–19, 117.

11. A. R. Gatrad, "Muslim Customs Surrounding Death, Bereavement, Postmortem, Examinations, and Organ Transplants," *BMJ* 309, no. 6943 (1994): 521.

12. Sachedina, 176. As Sachedina explains, this makes autopsies and post-mortem organ donations not illegal, but difficult to justify in Islamic biomedical ethics. He argues that they are possible for either determining the cause of death or, in the case of organ donation, possible through "arranging objectives in an ethical hierarchy—*qaida bab al-tazahum . . .*" in which saving another life can be prioritized.

13. Usually, the mourning period is observed by the family of the deceased and their community for forty days, 120 days, or other length of time, depending on the culture. Some cultures mark the one-year death anniversary by hosting a Qur'an recitation at the family's home.

14. Sachedina, 174–75.

15. In some cultures, including many Turkish and some South Asian cultures, it is not atypical for circumcision to take place sometime before the age of six, with much ceremony. Female circumcision is not sanctioned through Islamic scriptural sources, but sometimes it is practiced in the name of Islam or a culture that might be conflated with Islam. See Kecia Ali, *Sexual Ethics and Islam* (London: Oneworld, 2016), which contains a chapter on the subject.

16. Alison Shaw, "'They Say Islam Has a Solution for Everything, So Why Are There No Guidelines for This?' Ethical Dilemmas associated with the Births and Deaths of Infants with Fatal Abnormalities from a Small Sample of Pakistani Muslim Couples in Britain," *Bioethics* 26, no. 9 (November 2012): 491.

17. Vardit Rispler-Chaim, "The Right Not to Be Born: Abortion of the Disadvantaged Fetus in Contemporary Fatwas," *Muslim World* 89, no. 2 (April 1999): 130.

18. Alison Shaw, "Rituals of Infant Death: Defining Life and Islamic Personhood" *Bioethics* 28, no 2. (2014): 84–95, 88–89. Is it possible that this definition of legal personhood is a post-colonial, Western construct that is imported into Muslim practice? Rispler-Chaim says, and as several sources have attested, "in most of the Western world today personhood begins at birth." "The Right Not to Be Born," 130.

19. Shaw, "Why Are There No Guidelines for This?" 490.

20. Kathryn Kueny, *Conceiving Identities: Maternity in Medieval Muslim Discourse and Practice* (Albany: State University of New York Press, 2013), 9.

21. Omnia El Shakry, "Science: Medicalization and the Female Body," in *Encyclopedia of Women and Islamic Cultures*, ed. Suad Joseph (Leiden: E. J. Brill, 2006), 353–54;

Hibba Abugidieri, *Gender and the Making of Modern Medicine in Colonial Egypt* (London: Routledge, 2016), 116.

22. Da Costa, 115.

23. Ibid., 117.

24. Shaw, "Why Are There No Guidelines for This?" 491.

25. Ibid.

26. A. Lundqvist, T. Nilstun, and A. K. Dykes, "Neonatal End-of-Life Care in Sweden: The Views of Muslim Women," *Journal of Perinatal and Neonatal Nursing* 17, no. 1 (January–March 2003): 80–81.

27. Ibid., 80.

28. Ibid., 80.

29. F. Husain, "Ethical Dimensions of Non-Aggressive Fetal Management: A Muslim Perspective," *Seminars in Fetal and Neonatal Medicine* 13, no. 5 (October 2008): 323–24.

30. Alison Shaw, "Rituals of Infant Death: Defining Life and Islamic Personhood," *Bioethics* 28, no. 2 (2014): 85.

31. Shaw, "Why Are There No Guidelines for This?" 487.

32. Ibid., 487.

33. Ibid., 487.

34. Ibid., 487.

35. Ibid., 488.

36. Lundqvist and Dykes, 79.

37. Vardit Rispler-Chaim, *Islamic Medical Ethics in the Twentieth Century* (Leiden: E. J. Brill, 1993), 14.

38. Ibid., 14–15.

39. Ibid., 15.

40. Rispler-Chaim, "The Right Not to Be Born," 134–35.

41. Farhat Moazzam, *Bioethics and Organ Transplantation in a Muslim Society: A Study in Culture, Ethnography, and Religion* (Bloomington: Indiana University Press, 2016), 109–21.

42. Sherine Hamdy, *Our Bodies Belong to God: Organ Transplants, Islam, and the Struggle for Human Dignity in Egypt* (Berkeley: University of California Press, 2012), 36–37. In her work on organ transplantation in Egypt, Sherine Hamdy found that families trusted doctors to have adapted medical knowledge to the Egyptian Muslim case and often asked physicians their opinions on Islamic biomedical ethics questions.

6

A Muslim Neonatologist in a Canadian NICU

Juzer M. Tyebkhan

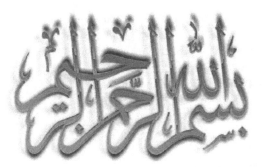

In the name of Al'laah, the most merciful, the most beneficent.

I offer this personal narrative of a Muslim neonatologist practicing in Edmonton, Canada, in the hope of providing some insight into what it means to Muslim families to have a baby in the neonatal intensive care unit (NICU). I had the opportunity to present this paper at the 2015 Gravens Conference in Florida and am honored that the organizers of the session "Spirituality in the NICU" felt that these reflections were worthy of inclusion in this collection.

I will begin by disclosing that I do not have qualifications in theology or philosophy, or any such field of study. I am a neonatologist who has a rather boring background of going from school to medical school to pediatric residency to neonatology—with no other careers or sidetracks. I must also be clear that my perspectives do not represent the viewpoints of all sects within the greater Muslim community, but rather reflect the beliefs and values of the Dawoodi Bohra Muslim community. I am the father of four beautiful children, who were fortunate enough to only enter the NICU to find their father, who was too often "still at work."

The Heritage of the Dawoodi Bohra Muslim Community

Perhaps it will help the reader if a few definitions are provided, as we begin. "Al-Islaam" is the name of the religion, and "Muslim" means a follower of this religion. All Muslims believe that Al'laah is the One Supreme Creator and that Mohammed[saw1] is Al'laah's Messenger. Al Qur'aan, the Divine Revelation of Al'laah, was given to Mohammed[saw].

To understand how a family from the Dawoodi Bohra community might feel about their baby in the NICU, and how their spiritual beliefs might affect that experience, a brief description of the community's spiritual heritage follows.[2] The relevance of this will be more obvious in later sections of this chapter.

The Dawoodi Bohra Muslims belong to the Shi'a Fatemi Tayyibi Dawoodi branch of the tree of al-Islam. This is shown diagrammatically with a brief explanation of each term:

Muslim   = the belief that Al'laah is the One Supreme Creator and that
                Mohammed[saw] is Al'laah's Messenger

↓

Shi'a   = the belief that Imaam 'Ali[as3] is Mohammed's[saw] successor

↓

Fatemi   = the belief that the Fatemi Imaams are the direct descendants and
                successors of Mohammed[saw] and 'Ali[as]. There is always one Imaam on
                Earth to lead Al'laah's mission.

↓

Tayyibi   = refers to the twenty-first Imaam, Tayyib[as]. Our belief is that His
                descendants have chosen to live in seclusion. The Imaams have ap-
                pointed the Da'i as their representative to guide their followers. There is
                always one Da'i present among the faithful, who functions as the vicege-
                rent of the Imaam.

↓

Dawoodi   = refers to the Da'i Syedna Dawood, during whose time as the Da'i, about four hundred years ago, the community became known by His name.

Bohra   = not a term that denotes an aspect of religious faith. Bohra means "trader," reflecting the main occupation of the community; to this day, it is the commonly used term that identifies the community. The largest populations of Dawoodi Bohras reside in India, Pakistan, Yemen, and East Africa. There are also significant numbers living in Europe, North America, South East Asia, and Australia. It is estimated that, worldwide, there are more than one million Dawoodi Bohras.

Our faith is that the chain of succession of the Imaams continues uninterrupted, from father to son, even while the Imaams are in seclusion. During this period of seclusion, the chain of succession of the Da'is also continues uninterrupted so that there is always one Da'i on this earth who guides our community. The Da'i is the spiritual link between the Dawoodi Bohras—via the Imaams, Ali[as], and the Prophet Mohammed[saw]—and Al'laah the Creator.

All Muslims believe that the Qur'aan was given to Mohammed[saw] by Divine Revelation. Mohammed[saw] thus became the custodian of the Divine Knowledge that reposes within the verses and words of the Qu'raan. The Dawoodi Bohras believe that the Da'i, by virtue of his spiritual link to Al'laah via the Imaams, Ali[as], and Mohammed[saw], is entrusted with the Divine Knowledge encompassed in Al'Qu'raan.

Today, the fifty-third Da'i, His Holiness Dr. Syedna Mufaddal Saifuddin, is our spiritual Father. Our faith is that He is the ultimate authority for all matters: religious, personal, material, and medical.

Islam, Health, and Healing

Islamic perspectives of health and healing can be gleaned from the following quotes:

- "And when I am sick, it is He (Al'laah) who cures." This Qur'aanic verse is ascribed to the Prophet Ibrahim[saw] (Abraham), and reminds us that health and healing are gifts from the Supreme Creator.
- "Avail of healing and medicine: Al'laah has not caused any illness to befall you, but has also created a cure for it." This is from the Hadith [Sacred Words] of the Prophet Mohammed[saw]. This teaching, to "avail of healing and medicine," makes it clear that it is not adequate to simply accept illness

and forgo attempts to regain health. This tenet of belief distinguishes Islam from other faiths that refuse modern medicine and treatments as a matter of religious principle.

- "Three things are essential for those who would become healers: piety towards Al'laah, the intention to always do good, and hard work." This is from the teachings of Imaam 'Ali[as]. I have reminded young friends within my community of this teaching when they ask me if they should or could become a doctor, and I encouraged them to reflect on these words as they consider why they wish to enter the healing profession. These words are potently re-energizing for those of us who work in the NICU, where exhaustion and burnout are not uncommon.

- "Those who work to heal the sick are only instruments of the Creator." Stated by Imaam Ja'far us Sadiq[as], these words serve to focus our purpose and goals as healers. Perhaps they also help us acknowledge our shortcomings and inadequacies in providing perfect health and healing to those in our care.

To relate these philosophical aspects of health and healing back to the spiritual heritage of the Dawoodi Bohras, described in the first section of this chapter, the reader is reminded that we consider the Da'i to be the ultimate authority for all matters: religious, personal, material, *and medical*. Today, when faced with critical illness, or when life-or-death decisions need to be made, the Dawoodi Bohras will ask the Da'i, His Holiness Dr. Syedna Mufaddal Saifuddin, for His prayers and His advice.

The Birth of a Muslim Baby

In anticipation of the baby's arrival, and in addition to the usual practical preparations, various religious and traditional observances occur during the months before the birth. The mother is encouraged to recite the Qur'aan, specifically the chapter of Mariyam (Mary), in which the birth of the Prophet 'Eesaa (Jesus) is narrated in detail. The recitation of the Qur'aan is not only a requirement for pregnant mothers; we are all expected to do so daily. This recitation is often done aloud, in melodic tones. Recent research that shows how prenatal auditory experiences prepare the child's neurological pathways of hearing makes this religious observance (i.e., the recitation of the Qur'aan during pregnancy) very intriguing to me as a neonatologist.

It is customary that the mother returns to her parents' house for the birth of the first child, although this doesn't mean that the child is born at home. The maternal grandmother-to-be often organizes a prayer meeting, with a celebratory

dinner to follow, for other women and daughters of the community, at the beginning of the ninth month, when the expectant mother comes back home. These
are not strict religious requirements, but rather are traditions that have the practical benefits of physical and emotional support for the mother during and after
the birth. They also allow the new mother to focus on feeding and looking after
the baby and to not have other responsibilities for the initial exhausting weeks.
Today, with families spread across the globe, it is not uncommon that the maternal grandmother travels to her daughter's house for the event.

At the time of birth, prayers are whispered into the child's ears, which include
the Adhaan (call to prayer) and various verses from the Qur'aan. The Bohra tradition is to name the child during the naming ceremony, which occurs on the
sixth day, and this is followed by the 'Aqiqa ceremony (see later). If the infant is
admitted to the NICU, these ceremonies might still be possible, with some crea-
tivity and openness on the part of the NICU.

So, how can the NICU facilitate these important ceremonies around the time
of birth of a Dawoodi Bohra Muslim baby? We know that many fathers and
relatives who accompany the infant to the NICU are scared to touch or even
come close to the child, let alone ask if they can hold the child to recite prayers
into his or her ears. However, if NICU personnel ask them if they would like
to do this, the answer is usually, "Yes, but how can I?" Working out how the father (often the person who will recite these prayers) can hold his baby soon after
NICU admission, or guiding him to bend over the cot and whisper into his baby's
ears, makes this an easily achieved milestone for both father and baby.

The Dawoodi Bohra tradition is to ask His Holiness to choose the child's
name, and this may have been done during the pregnancy or may be requested
once the child is born. As mentioned previously, the naming ceremony occurs
on the sixth day, and it is customary for the child's paternal aunt to perform this
ceremony, which involves holding the child on her lap, dressing him or her in a
white tunic and cap, reciting the Adhaan and verses from the Qur'aan into the
child's ears, and, finally, whispering the name into his or her ears. This ceremony
is a celebratory occasion for family and friends, and, in recent times, "Who can
guess the baby's name?" has also become part of the festivities, with a gift expected by whoever guessed correctly.

The naming ceremony can be also done on a smaller scale if the child is in the
hospital. For the few minutes that it takes for this naming ceremony, it should be
possible to be flexible with NICU visiting rules, so that at least the paternal aunt
can come in with the parents if space is extremely limited and if moving to a private
room, where more family could be accommodated, is not possible. NICUs that are
adept at helping parents hold and cuddle babies on varying degrees of life support
technology could probably help the aunt hold the child on her lap, although this
may take some preplanning so that she knows what to expect. If this isn't possible,

then any of us can easily help the aunt bend over the bed so that she is nearer the child's head. If practical to do so, she may appreciate help with putting on the white cotton tunic, but again, if this isn't possible, the tunic can simply be placed on the child's trunk. The prayers that are recited into the baby's ears take only a few minutes, after which the appropriate boxes on hospital forms that have probably been highlighted as "incomplete" can be filled in to satisfy hospital administration.

The naming ceremony is followed by the 'Aqiqa, which occurs either on day seven, fourteen, or twenty-one. The relative of honor for this event is the maternal uncle; it is interesting that both sides of the family are given specific roles in these birth-related celebrations. At the 'Aqiqa, the uncle holds the child on his lap while the child's head is shaved. This does become a little more complicated than the naming ceremony because it may be technically difficult to do this if the child is on life support therapies. However, for the infant in the NICU who is relatively well, it may just require some creative thinking on our part to facilitate this practice. The uncle does not shave the hair; his role is simply to hold the child. In countries such as India, a barber may come to do this, or a member of the local Bohra community may have taken on this task. Again, with preplanning, it may be possible to arrange for the 'Aqiqa in the NICU. A member of the staff, such as a neonatologist, nurse practitioner, or the intravenous (IV) team—who are likely comfortable with shaving infants' hair to find IV sites—could become part of the celebration and officiate in this role, if hospital rules and regulations do not allow a non–staff member to do this. In the event that the 'Aqiqa cannot be performed, it is deferred until the child reaches adulthood.

How Neonatal Intensive Care Unit Admission Can Affect the Dawoodi Bohra Muslim Family

Breastfeeding and Breast Milk

Breastfeeding is an important mothering role that is emphasized by Islamic teachings. The Qur'aan states that a child should be breastfed for up to two years[4]; another verse states that "the carrying of the child and the weaning is (for a period) of thirty months."[5] Breastfeeding mothers are not expected to fast during the holy month of Ramadaan if fasting adversely affects breastfeeding. Muslim mothers may, however, have some reservations about breastfeeding in the NICU if there is limited privacy (see later discussion of Hijaab and Purdah).

Bohra Muslim mothers will in all likelihood appreciate the expertise of NICU staff with respect to breastfeeding and lactation assistance. However, the topic of donor breast milk needs some elaboration because this will not be acceptable to Dawoodi Bohra Muslim families, unless the donor is known to them. Breast milk is considered to create kinship between the mother who provides the milk and all the children who receive her milk, regardless of whether the milk is obtained by suckling at the breast or by expression and then fed to the infant. This milk kinship means that all the children who receive the milk of one mother are now siblings and cannot marry one another. In fact, some families will formally create this close relationship with another family by having two lactating mothers (i.e., one of each family) breastfeed the other's baby. This is not a very common practice today, but I mention this to illustrate the significance of breast milk and the kinship that it confers.

Thus, donor milk, especially pooled donor milk, will not be acceptable to Bohra families. The reader is reminded that the authority for religious and worldly matters, for the Dawoodi Bohras, is the Da'i. The opinions of other Muslim scholars—that permit donor milk for infants in the NICU[6]—do not therefore carry similar authority, and these publications should not be used to convince Bohra families to accept this form of nutrition. However, the milk of another known Dawoodi Bohra or Muslim mother may be acceptable because the milk-mother and milk-siblings would be known to both donor and recipient families. Although it is not usual practice in the Edmonton NICUs to have "designated milk donation," we have had instances where families—both Muslim and non-Muslim—have stated their preference for this, and the NICU now makes allowances for this.

The reader may wonder why we in Edmonton have made allowances for designated milk donors that include a requirement for the parents to sign a document stating that this is their individual choice. We realized some years ago that, occasionally, mothers brought in "pumped breast milk" that was not their own but instead a relative's or friend's milk. They then labeled and froze it as their own milk so that it would be used for their infant, although they were simultaneously asking for lactation support because they had almost no milk themselves. Rather than continuing the pretense of this situation, we have now accepted this uncommon practice so that these infants can receive breast milk without their families needing to be secretive. Discussing "designated milk donation" may, therefore, be a mechanism by which the benefits of breast milk can be provided to infants whose families would otherwise opt for formula when the mother does not have sufficient milk herself.

Medical Treatments that May Be Considered
Haraam (Forbidden)

There may be instances in which routine treatments need discussion and some flexibility on our parts. Islam strictly forbids the consumption of pig-derived products in any form and of alcohol. These may be either the source (e.g., porcine surfactant) or components of prescribed treatments. In most cases, patients and families are unlikely to know the sources and components of their treatments and drugs, unless they ask. However, for those with a deep religious faith, subsequent knowledge that something forbidden was ingested, even unintentionally, may become a source of personal distress. In the NICU, this angst may contribute to the overall stress experienced by parents. In this section, I would like the reader to consider (1) the significance to the family of providing a treatment or intervention for their infant without informing them of details that may have personal meaning to them, and (2) the options that are possible if a family has reservations about a suggested treatment plan.

Surfactants available for clinical use are either bovine-derived or porcine-derived.[7] Most NICUs use one formulation of surfactant, and, since this is now a standard treatment for respiratory distress of the preterm infant, the NICU's usual surfactant is likely to be given without formal consent; at times, parents are simply informed after the event. Although there is some urgency to treat respiratory distress, surfactant does not usually have to be administered within minutes of birth.

For Muslim babies, if given a choice, their families will opt for a bovine-derived surfactant. Can a NICU that has chosen a porcine surfactant as the usual treatment consider (1) discussing this treatment with family that are present and (2) having available a bovine surfactant to use for these infants? The second suggestion, to have a different surfactant available, may create administrative discontent, but this should not deter us from providing an equally effective treatment that is more acceptable to the family and that may alleviate some of their distress.

Pig-derived products are also part of some of the special elemental formulas used for feeding babies who have had intestinal complications. There are options that are free of porcine enzymes; again, this may require the NICU to have available the formula that would be more acceptable to Muslim families. A similar situation may arise with respect to the use of alcohol in medications. Although many pediatric formulations now avoid using alcohol, those that contain alcohol would likely not be acceptable to the Muslim family. Again, this is a situation in which frank discussion with the family may lead to a mutually acceptable alternative.

How the Dawoodi Bohra Community Deals with Life-or-Death Decisions

As mentioned in the first section of this chapter, the Dawoodi Bohra faith is that the Da'i—who today is His Holiness Dr. Syedna Mufaddal Saifuddin—is the ultimate authority for all matters: religious, personal, material, and medical. The Dawoodi Bohra's faith is that the advice provided by His Holiness is divinely guided as a result of His spiritual link with Al'laah the Creator.

When faced with life-or-death situations related to pregnancy and the new-born, a Dawoodi Bohra family will present the situation to His Holiness, together with the medical details and treatment options their doctors have discussed with them, and they will ask for His prayers and His direction. The direction He gives for treatment is then accepted as the correct decision for that infant and family and does not need further deliberation or debate.

I have been privileged to have been part of some of these difficult situations, when Dawoodi Bohra families around the world have asked for help in presenting to His Holiness the specifics of their child's condition and the treatment recommendations and options of the specialists involved. Over the years, these have included infants with lethal conditions diagnosed in pregnancy, children with severe congenital anomalies, those with complex illnesses that have uncertain outcomes after prolonged NICU treatment, and families considering options for withdrawing life support treatments. Given current electronic communication channels, the case can be presented to the administrative offices of His Holiness within a very short time span.

It is important to point out that each situation is considered individually and that the guidance provided for one child will not necessarily be the same as that for another with a similar condition. It is certainly not the case that the withdrawal of life support treatment would never be permitted, or that all possible life-saving treatments must be attempted regardless of complications. For some infants, the direction may be to follow the recommended plan of the specialists; for example, this may be the case for those who are critically ill but whose treatment plan is relatively straightforward, albeit complex. For children whose condition is not rapidly lethal but whose experience of life is significantly different from that of their age-equivalent peers, there may be several reports presented to His Holiness over time, and treatment plans may change with time, given the changing status of the child. These include conditions such as neurodegenerative diseases, complex congenital heart disease, and Trisomies 13 and 18.

The advice and guidance of His Holiness in these situations are accompanied by His prayers and blessings, which provide comfort and solace for Bohra families during these difficult situations. At times, families of other faiths, including Muslims from other communities, approach His Holiness for His prayers and for guidance regarding critical illness in their families. Blessings and advice are bestowed on these families, with similar fatherly concern as when this is provided to Bohra families.

When a Baby Dies

The death of a Muslim baby may require some adjustment of the routines of North American hospitals and NICUs in order to help the family with the religious rites associated with this.

In general, autopsy is not permitted; however, for infants who are critically ill, it may be acceptable to some families if investigations such as muscle or tissue biopsy are done before the child dies rather than post mortem. If time permits, talking to the family while there is still time for these procedures may enable them to be done rather than to be declined after the child dies.

When death is imminent, the Bohra Muslim family will ask the Aamil (the local priest of the congregation) to officiate at the prayers recited at this time. The bed (or the infant) should be turned to face Makkah, such that the infant's feet are pointing in that direction. After the child passes away, the limbs should be positioned extended, and the body should not be interfered with in any way; for example, it is not acceptable to cut a lock of the child's hair as a memento. The body will be ritually bathed by members of the community before burial; thus, it is not necessary for NICU staff to do so. Neither is it the practice to clothe the baby in new or personal clothing; Islamic funeral rites require that the body is bathed, shrouded in unstitched white cotton, and then buried.

Islamic teachings are that the body should be buried as soon as possible, meaning that the relevant paperwork needs to be completed so that the family can make funeral arrangements. From the perspective of the infant who dies in the NICU, this requires the availability of medical staff to sign death certificates and hospital administration to complete documentation that will allow the body to be released, even when death occurs outside of "business" hours. Muslim families (as well as others who require burial as soon as possible) reluctantly accept having to wait until Monday morning should the infant die over the weekend because they may have no choice in the matter. However, it seems somewhat illogical that intensive care and emergency services function around the clock, yet simple clerical work that would allow the family some relief from the stress of their child's final illness can only be provided during office hours. I leave this for the reader to contemplate.

Helping Muslim Families in the Neonatal Intensive Care Unit

How can NICU staff help a Muslim family so that their baby's NICU journey aligns with the expected journey of a (Dawoodi Bohra) Muslim baby who did not need NICU admission? This statement should probably be expanded to "How can the NICU staff help *every* family so that their baby's NICU journey aligns with the expected journey of a baby who did not need NICU admission?" Although there are many aspects that could be discussed, and each family may have individual preferences for what they consider most relevant, for brevity I will focus on (1) space for parents and privacy, (2) meals, and (3) prayer as it relates to the Dawoodi Bohra Muslim family.

Space for Parents and Privacy

We know that the active participation of parents in the infant's care leads to many improved outcomes, including a reduced length of stay in the NICU.[8,9] NICUs are now designed or renovated so that there is adequate space for parents to live with their infant and to be part of the caregiving, yet also space for their privacy.

In this respect, the Muslim mother may prefer more privacy than is currently possible at many NICU bedsides, given the Islamic tenet of "Hijaab" (also known as "Purdah"). This is the principle that a woman's physical beauty is private, not to be shown to men to whom she is not closely related, as is evident in the traditional clothing that Muslim women wear outside the house. Dawoodi Bohra women wear a two-piece outfit called the "rida," which consists of a full-length skirt and an upper cape that fits over the head and upper body. (At home, the upper cape is exchanged for a headscarf.) The rida may be of any color and is often enhanced with embroidery or lace; it thus differs from the burqas or chadors worn by other Muslim women, which are usually plain and of dark colors. The two-piece garment makes breastfeeding relatively easy when the mother is out of the house because the infant can be easily brought to the breast under the top part of the rida, while the mother herself remains completely covered. In the NICU, however, where observation of the infant during skin-to-skin care and breastfeeding may be required, some mothers may be reluctant to do this unless there is a guarantee of privacy such as within a single room or a space with fixed floor-to-ceiling partitions. As NICUs implement single-family-room design, it is likely that Muslim mothers will be more comfortable to breastfeed and provide skin-to-skin care in the unit.

Meals

The availability in the hospital of nutritious meals for parents is a factor that can make it easier for them to stay in the NICU to help look after their infant for an extended period of time. Many hospitals have limited options of food for purchase; for those who have dietary restrictions, the choice is even more limited. As already mentioned, pig-derived products are not permitted. In addition, only meat that is halal will be eaten by observant Muslims; *halal* means that the animal has been slaughtered according to religious law. Halal meat is available in the majority of larger cities in North America, and hospitals that serve the Muslim population could be encouraged to serve halal options. As a Muslim who has often had to eat at hospital cafeterias, I am often both amused and disappointed with the "vegetarian" options, which are the next best option when halal is not available. The choice is usually between fries, onion rings, soggy salad, fruit, or pasta drowned in processed, melted cheese—a selection that is hardly likely to encourage parents to stay with their infants over mealtimes for several days or weeks.

It has also been suggested that NICUs should provide parental meals without charge. Since the optimal care of the newborn infant requires the presence of a parent as the primary caregiver, the NICU patient is more correctly the dyad of infant plus parent. In Edmonton, our NICU-FACT (Family Advisory Care Team) has identified "meals for NICU parents" as a project for their wish list. Whether other NICUs decide to pursue free meals for parents or not, the goal of facilitating parental participation in their infant's care is certainly one for all NICUs. Ensuring that food of sufficient variety, quality, palatability, and religious acceptability is available could be accomplished without significant administrative effort.

Prayer

Five prayers each day are obligatory for all Muslims, although there is a special dispensation for postpartum mothers for the first forty days after delivery. Fathers and other family members may wish to pray at the prescribed times, which are dependent on the timing of sunrise and sunset and so change as the length of the day varies with the seasons. The admission of an infant to the NICU itself may be a factor for some Muslim families to be more observant of the daily prayers. It may be important for some families that case conferences and other meetings are arranged so that they don't overlap with prayer time; this is more relevant for the sunset prayer, for which the prescribed time span is relatively short.

If space for prayer is available in or near the NICU, this may also facilitate family presence and participation in infant care. A corner of the NICU's family lounge could be screened off for this purpose; a strictly private space is not always essential. Although most smartphones are now equipped with a compass that can indicate the direction of Makkah, a sign in the prayer area showing this direction—toward which Muslims pray—will be sincerely appreciated.

Conclusion

I have attempted to describe my personal thoughts about the NICU experience for Muslim families and how our religious traditions and requirements might affect that experience. As stated in the introduction, this is a personal viewpoint I give as a Dawoodi Bohra Muslim neonatologist practicing in Canada, and not as an authority on Islamic religious law. However, many of the topics I have described will likely be applicable to Muslim families of other denominations. These include the desire for alternatives to alcohol- and porcine-derived treatments or medications and the reluctance to use banked breast milk because of kinship issues. Declining autopsy and the requirement for prompt burial would be a common wish for most Muslim families. With respect to encouraging parental participation in their infant's care, privacy for skin-to-skin treatments, space for prayer, and halal-friendly meals would help many Muslim families, not just the Bohra family.

I also wish to be clear that each Dawoodi Bohra family is unique, with medically related decision making influenced by individual features of each family; this narrative should not be taken as a prescription that applies to all.

Therefore, I end this chapter by reflecting on my twenty-plus years of working in the NICU, attempting to help infants and families of many faith-based backgrounds and from different religious traditions. Each family has taught me that what is most significant and meaningful for them is unique and highly individual, and in many cases, was not what I would have guessed. In conclusion, I leave the reader with the following thought:

Helping a Dawoodi Bohra Muslim family when their baby is in the NICU, so that religious observances and traditions can be fulfilled while their infant is treated, is no different than helping families of other faiths. Quite simply, just ask:

- "What is important for you?" and
- "How can we help you?"

And then, be creative as you try to provide that help.

With that, I leave you with the traditional Muslim greeting of Welcome and Farewell: السلام عليكم "As-salaamo alaykum" (Peace be upon you).

Notes

1. The superscript SAW, written after the names of the Prophets Ibrahim and Mohammed, means "Peace Be upon Him and upon His Progeny." The letters SAW denote the Arabic version of this invocation.
2. Al-Da'i Al-Fatemi Syedna Mohammed Burhanuddin, *An Illustrated Biography* (London: Al-Jamea-tus-Saifiyah Trust, 2001), distributed by Oxford University Press).
3. The superscript AS, after the names of 'Ali and the Imaams, means "Peace Be upon Him."
4. Al-Qur'aan: Suraa 2:322.
5. Ibid., 46:15.
6. Afif El-Khuffash and Sharon Unger, "The Concept of Milk Kinship in Islam: Issues Raised when Offering Preterm Infants of Muslim Families Donor Human Milk," *Journal of Human Lactation* 28 (2012): 125–27.
7. Smeeta Sardesai et al., "Evolution of Surfactant Therapy for Respiratory Distress Syndrome: Past, Present, and Future," *Pediatric Research* 81, no 1–2 (January 2017): 240–48.
8. Kathrine Leigh Peters et al., "Improvement of Short- and Long-Term Outcomes for Very Low Birth Weight Infants: Edmonton NIDCAP Trial," *Pediatrics* 124 (2009): 1009–20.
9. Annica Örtenstrand et al., "The Stockholm Neonatal Family Centered Care Study: Effects on Length of Stay and Infant Morbidity," *Pediatrics* 125 (2010): e278–85.

7

Shiva's Babies

Hindu Perspectives on the Treatment of High-Risk Newborn Infants

Swasti Bhattacharyya

In our current global context, local communities are increasingly diverse. This diversity is present in large metropolitan areas and in small, rural towns. Across the United States and the world, more cities have English, German, Guatemalan, Hmong, and Sudanese—among many others—living side by side. Buddhist and Hindu temples are within blocks of synagogues, mosques, and countless churches. Understanding this religious and cultural diversity has important implications for those working in health care.

It is not reasonable to expect healthcare providers to know the religious and cultural ideologies of all their patients and families, or to know all the complexities that make up their lives. However, being sensitive to the fact that these differences exist and attentive to addressing the needs of each individual is necessary for health care to be competent. When effective health care is delivered with *cultural humility*, the results are remarkable.[1] Therefore, I begin this chapter by establishing what cultural humility means. Then, I present six characteristics common to many perspectives grounded in Hindu traditions. Finally, through the voices of adult residents of the United States who self-identify as Hindu, I explore how these characteristically Hindu attitudes and beliefs might come into play for families and healthcare providers in the neonatal intensive care unit (NICU).

Healthcare professionals understand the language of proficiency and competency. We are forever checking off the boxes, demonstrating that we indeed know how to do our jobs and can do them very well, even excellently. However, I begin this chapter with a discussion of *cultural humility*,[2] as opposed to cultural *competency*, because arriving at an appropriate response to difference is not about acquiring knowledge of principles or propositions (competency). Rather, cultural humility focuses on how we prepare ourselves to listen so that we can hear the hopes, fears, and needs of our patients and their families. In the context of competency, detached mastery of a finite body of knowledge can be an end in and of itself. A nurse could learn fifty important teachings of Hinduism. Knowing this and simply applying it uniformly to all patients—all families, in the case of the NICU—assumed to be Hindu would not necessarily enhance care. However, in the context of cultural humility, we learn about particular Hindu ideas or beliefs for the sake of opening our minds and thereby increasing our capacity to understand. With an open mind, perhaps we as healthcare providers will be more receptive to different possibilities and able to hear new questions and concerns voiced by our patients and their families.

Cultural humility takes into account the complex, ever-changing realities of life. It encourages healthcare providers to have an attitude of commitment and active engagement in a lifelong process of learning—a commitment to learning from patients, community members, and colleagues. According to Foronda et al., cultural humility "incorporates a lifelong commitment to self-evaluation and critique, to redressing the power imbalances in the physician-patient dynamic, and to developing mutually beneficial and non-paternalistic partnerships with communities on behalf of individuals and defined populations." They go on to say that it is

> a process of openness, self-awareness, being egoless, and incorporating self-reflection and critique after willingly interacting with diverse individuals. The results of achieving cultural humility are mutual empowerment, respect, partnerships, optimal care, and lifelong learning.[3]

As this definition indicates, cultural humility is an ever-evolving process, not something to be completed. It begins with each of us becoming more aware of who we are and more open to seeing others for who they are.

As healthcare providers, we need to know ourselves. Being aware of our own worldview enables us to understand that we indeed see the world from a particular perspective. This awareness, coupled with an attitude of humility, can increase our ability to hear and understand others. Once a physician knows who she is, and she develops the skills of mindfully listening (i.e., listening for understanding, not to label or categorize), she will be a physician more capable of hearing what her patient and the family are saying. In hearing, she will be better able to address the needs that her patient (or in the case of an infant, the family) expresses.

While cultural competency focuses on skills and gathering information about different religions and cultures, cultural humility "implies one must strive for learning at the highest level of learning: that of transformation."[4] Cultural humility is not a skill to be mastered, but rather is a way of being that begins with self-awareness. It allows us to let our perspectives recede so that we can see and assess the patient before us. One of the mantras in nursing school was to "always look at the patient." We were continually told, "Don't rely on monitors, look at the patient and assess." The same is true in this context.

All Hindus, all Buddhists, or all Christians do not believe the same thing. Even folks within the same family have different expressions and experiences of their culture and faith. Having cultural humility means we walk into a patient's room and listen as they describe and define themselves (or as the infant's family expresses these things). We pay close attention, keep an open mind, and do not presume. Doing this allows us to better assess our patients and their situation. The more accurate our assessment, the more effective our responses and treatments will be. It is into this atmosphere that I bring a discussion of different Hindu ideas. It is helpful to learn about other traditions because this knowledge exposes us to different ideas and ways of thinking so that when we encounter our patients, we can work together through the implications of their or their families' worldviews and current situation. When we combine cultural humility with medical expertise, we are able to provide excellent and effective care.

Characteristics of Hindu Thought

The idea that nothing is monolithic is true for all religious traditions; diversity abounds within Buddhism, Christianity, and Judaism, among others. The fact that this plurality of thought is also present in Hinduism is not unique. However, the term *Hinduism* itself is foreign, historically late, disputed, and complicated. The term was used to identify indigenous people living east of the Indus River (currently in Pakistan, west of India) who were not Jewish, Christian, or Muslim. The origins of the term *Hindu* did not refer to a particular people, belief, or ideology. Therefore, it is not surprising that within Hindu traditions, no one deity, text, or leader is considered authoritative for all groups that identify as Hindu. There is also no single common belief that unites all the groups or peoples who lay claim to the term *Hindu* or *Hinduism*. In addition, like the languages of other traditional cultures, Sanskrit, an ancient language of India, does not have a word for *religion*; there is no clear distinction between religion and life. So, when listening to those speaking within Hindu traditions, one often encounters fluidity between the concepts of religion, culture, and life. Hindu traditions include differing, even contradictory, perspectives, and there is an ability to hold a great deal of ambiguity. This very mercurial nature is a characteristic of traditions that fall within what we call Hinduism.

Keeping this flexibility in mind, there are shared characteristics that underlie a number of the worldviews that fall within Hinduism, many of which are especially important in the NICU and hospital setting. Of the many characteristics,

I draw out the following: (1) the underlying unity of all life, (2) the centrality of society, (3) dharma, (4) the multivalent nature of Hindu traditions and beliefs, (5) karma, and (6) ahimsa. Again, while not universal, these six characteristics often play an instructive role for individuals with worldviews grounded in Hindu traditions.[5] After explaining each of these characteristics, I discuss them within the context of the NICU. Again, my hope is that this discussion provides insights for healthcare providers as they interact with families in the NICU and throughout the hospital.

A foundational metaphysical understanding of reality present in many worldviews grounded in Hinduism is the idea that there is an underlying unity of all life: there is an inseparable interconnectedness among everything. Brahman is the creator and the essence of everything. Ultimately, there is no distinction between Brahman and creation. There is also no distinction between Brahman and the soul or self, "Atman." While monotheistic traditions usually draw a distinction between God, the creator, and that which is created, human beings and the world, Advaita Vedanta philosophy, described here, does not. This unity is expressed in a number of formative texts:

> His mouth became Brahmin; his arms were made into the Warrior, his thighs the People, and from his feet the Servants were born. The moon was born from his mind; from his eye the sun was born. Indra and Agni came from his mouth, and from his vital breath the Wind was born. From his navel the middle realm of space arose; from his head the sky evolved. From his two feet came the earth, and the quarters of the sky from his ear. . . .[6]

This *Rig Vedic* text establishes that everything—humans, the caste system, the world, and universe—all originate from one entity: Brahman. The *Upanishads* also reflect this notion that Brahman is everything:

> In Him alone, as he shines, do all things reflect; this world radiates with his light. Brahman alone here extends to the east; brahman, to the west; it alone, to the south to the north, it alone extends above and below; it is brahman alone that extends over this whole universe, up to its widest extent.[7]

These are just two examples among countless texts that establish an underlying unity between all of creation and Brahman, ultimate reality.

Reiterating this unity, Shankara, the famous eighth-century Vedanta philosopher, writes:

> [36]I am verily that Supreme Brahman, which is eternal, stainless, and free; which is One, indivisible and nondual; and which is of the nature of Bliss, Truth,

Knowledge, and Infinity. . . . [38]Sitting in a solitary place, freeing the mind from desires, and controlling the senses, meditate with unswerving attention on Infinite Atman, which is One without a second. . . . [40]He who has attained the Supreme Goal discards all such objects as name and form, and dwells as the embodiment of Infinite Consciousness and Bliss.[8]

According to Shankara, the real, Brahman, is an indivisible Reality. This belief in the underlying unity of all reality is a thread found running through many worldviews grounded within Hinduism.

From this first characteristic, underlying unity of all life, flow several others, namely the centrality of society and dharma. When a person's worldview is grounded in an idea that everything is ultimately one reality, then it follows that a person may see himself, his role, in the context of a larger society. Rather than seeing and experiencing the self as an independent, autonomous individual, many people operating out of Hindu worldviews often begin with a more communal sense of identity and responsibility.

When speaking of Hinduism, many are familiar with the term "caste system"— the stratified nature of society. There are four traditional castes (with multiple sub-casts in-between) and each is connected to important roles that uphold and contribute to the success of society. In addition, traditional Hinduism highlights four *asramas*, or stages of life. These acknowledge the different stages individuals usually go through from birth through old age. According to the *Laws of Manu*, the householder stage is one of the most important:

> Just as all living creatures depend on air in order to live, so do members of the other stages of life subsist by depending on householders. Since people in the other three stages of life are supported every day by the knowledge and the food of the householder, the householder stage of life is the best.[9]

The householder, the stage of life in which a person has a family and establishes a career, is that of the person who supports and sustains society.[10] The observant householder realizes both the philosophical and actual interdependence of all. The caste system and stages of life are both interwoven into an understanding that reality is ultimately unified; they support the second characteristic of Hindu thought, the centrality of society.

In the United States, questions regarding what a person ought to do are often legal and individual: "What are my rights?" or "How might I benefit?" Rather than focusing on a person's individual rights or how a person can bring benefit to himself, a person operating out of Hindu worldviews will often consider his course of action within the context of the needs of the family and society. S. Radhakrishnan (Indian philosopher and statesman who was the first Vice

President and second President of India) emphasizes the centrality of society when he says:

> Human society is an organic whole, the parts of which are naturally dependent in such a way that each part in fulfilling its distinctive function conditions the fulfillment of function by the rest, and is in turn conditioned by the fulfillment of its function by the rest. In this sense the whole is present in each part, while each part is indispensable to the whole.[11]

When a person begins with the assumption that all of society is interdependent, and individuals have their standing because of their place within their family and society, then it often follows that this person will consider the needs of society as he makes personal decisions.

As a person considers her role in society and her stage of life, all this is embedded in the term *dharma*. Dharma is a difficult word to translate. This third characteristic is a central concept in Hindu traditions, but one that is context specific and very malleable. According the Monier-Williams *Sanskrit-English Dictionary*, "dharma" means, "That which is established or firm, steadfast, decree, statute, ordinance, law; usage, practice, customary observance or prescribed conduct, duty; right, justice (often as a synonym of punishment); virtue, morality, religion, religious merit, good works."[12] These definitions are indicative of just how diverse and mercurial the term *dharma* is.

Ultimately, for my purpose here, dharma refers to some sort of action, to prescribed behavior, or to the decisions, roles, and behaviors of individuals and groups. In the *Bhagavad Gita*, the God Krishna tells Arjuna, a great warrior,

> Look to your Law [dharma] and do not waver, for there is nothing more salutary for a baron than a war that is lawful. . . . Or suppose you will not engage in this lawful war: then you give up your Law [dharma] and honor, and incur guilt.[13]

As a warrior, Arjuna's dharma is to fight in this war that will bring peace and justice. If he were to refuse to fight, he would shirk his responsibilities, forfeit his honor, and incur the guilt of his nonaction. As a member of a family and community, each individual has a particular dharma, or particular roles and responsibilities. However, dharma is not an abstract universal principle; it is a term that ultimately relates in some manner to action or behavior. Dharma is more of a guideline that shifts and adjusts to the particular situation. Within society, each caste member has specific duties, and each stage of life does as well. So what might be "right" in one instance might not be so in another context. In a discussion on European philosophical ideas of virtue as opposed to those within Hinduism,

A. K. Ramanujan, an Indian poet and literary scholar, highlights the context-sensitive nature of dharma. Ramanujan indicates that the German philosopher Georg Wilhelm Friedrich Hegel may say "bravery is a virtue," but Ramanujan argues that, for Hindus, "Bravery is a virtue of the Kashatryas [warriors]." So, within these worldviews, virtue, duty, and how a person ought to act, or dharma, is often context specific.

Tightly interwoven with dharma is a notion of "nonattachment." Again, Krishna explains to Arjuna,

> Your entitlement is only to the rite, not ever at all to its fruits. Be not motivated by the fruits of acts, but also do not purposely seek to avoid acting. Abandon self-interest, Dhanamjaya [Arjuna], and perform the acts while applying this singlemindedness. Remain equable in success and failure. . . .[14]

A person is to perform his duty to the best of his ability, and then "let go," not be tied to the fruits, the successes or failures.

When considering Hindu ethics, dharma inevitably comes into the discussion. It is a central concept for many people operating out of Hindu worldviews. However, we must keep in mind that dharma, while tightly woven throughout Hindu worldviews, is neither absolute nor monolithic. It highlights the roles and duties of all within society, and these change depending on the situation. A son's duty to his mother is one thing. This same son has different duties and responsibilities to his partner, his children, and his colleagues.

This complicated, multi-layered understanding of dharma coincides with the fourth characteristic: the multivalent nature of traditions within Hinduism. Though each individual may have a particular dharma, what one person ought to do in a particular situation may not be the same for another. Though the Ultimate Reality is one, it is understood and discussed in many ways. Radhakrishnan describes it this way:

> A Hindu thinker readily admits other points of view than his own and considers them to be just as worthy of attention. After all, if the whole race of man, in every land, of every colour, and every stage of culture, is the offspring of God, then we must admit that, in the vast compass of his providence, all are being trained by his wisdom and supported by his love to reach within the limits of their powers a knowledge of the Supreme.[15]

Rather than grasping for absolutes, many within Hindu traditions carefully consider their roles and responsibilities and the particulars of the situation as they attempt to determine the best course of action. The flexibility of a person's dharma reflects the complexity of reality.

The multivalent nature of Hindu traditions does not establish clear, consistent, all-encompassing Philosophical treatises clearly declaring proper ethical behavior. However, Hindus are concerned with how individuals ought to act. Reflective of this, dharma implies movement toward order and sense of purpose. Each person is called to do her or his best toward that end. According to the *Bhagavad Gita*, it is better "to perform one's own duty (dharma) imperfectly than to perform the duty of another perfectly. Better to carry out one's own duty, even unto death, for to follow another's duty is perilous."[16] This flexibility might lead some to the conclusion that everything is relative or that there are no boundaries or limitations to human actions. Or it may lead others to assume that those within Hinduism are indifferent, defeatist, or have an "anything goes" attitude. However, S. Radhakrishnan explained it well when he said, "Hinduism does not mistake tolerance for indifference. It affirms that while all revelations refer to reality, they are not equally true to it."[17]

Traditions operating within Hindu worldviews are not indifferent. While the great deal of flexibility allowed within these traditions can lead to an idea that "anything goes," the fifth characteristic of Hindu thought, karma, puts this to rest. The law of karma holds everyone ultimately responsible for their actions. Be it in this life or the next, no one can avoid the consequences of his or her actions. Karma is neither fatalistic nor negative. Karma simply means "action." According to the *Bhagavad Gita*, "Indeed, no one can exist, even for a moment, without doing some action. Everyone is forced to work, helplessly driven by the forces born of nature."[18] Everyone, by virtue of being alive, cannot help but act. All action, be it past, present, or future, is inextricably tied to consequences. So, according to the law of karma, everyone reaps the fruits of their actions.

Though a person's past action, karma, may influence the person's current state, karma does not determine the person's current mode of action. While karma may determine the cards we hold in our hand, it does not determine how we play them: it does not make us powerless over the present or future. Each of us is free to play the hand as we see fit. Ultimately, the theory of karma calls individuals to a high level of responsibility; we are to act, and we are held responsible for the consequences of our actions (either in this life or the next).

When considering action—karma, dharma, and the other three characteristics of Hindu thought discussed earlier—a sixth underlying principle often comes into play: a commitment to "ahimsa." Ahimsa means "no harm" or "nonviolence." In a bioethical context, it can suggest principles of nonmaleficence and beneficence.[19] If one believes in an underlying unity of all life, in dharma, and in karma, then a commitment to ahimsa can be a logical expression. According to M. K. Gandhi,

> Attacking an individual, even an enemy, is tantamount to resisting and attacking oneself. For we are all tarred with the same brush, and are children

of one and the same Creator, and as such the divine powers within us are infinite. To slight a single human being is to slight those divine powers, and thus to
harm not only that being but with him the whole world.[20]

Gandhi grounds his argument for ahimsa in his belief in the underlying unity
of all life. Also, when acting with ahimsa (nonmaleficence and beneficence),
dharma can be fulfilled and the good of society served.

Worldviews grounded in Hinduism acknowledge the diversity of norms,
values, life experiences, and situations. These worldviews are not static or absolute: there is a recognition that life is complex and ever changing. No one text, law,
ideology, or philosophy can fully capture it. Thus, though the six characteristics
highlighted earlier may be foundational for those operating within Hinduism,
they all remain malleable as they are interpreted and applied. This ability to respond to the particulars of a situation, and the ability to embrace a great deal of
ambiguity, provides fertile ground in which to explore the complexities of life.

Application of Hindu Characteristics to the Neonatal
Intensive Care Unit

The previous discussion is not provided so that healthcare professionals might
have a template into which they can put patients and their families; doing so
could be disastrous. Rather, it is provided so that readers are introduced to particular vocabulary and ideas that can provide a glimpse into the worldviews of
some patients and families. As previously mentioned, the six characteristics of
Hindu thought are not all-encompassing, universally interpreted, or absolute.
Nevertheless, they are often reflected in Hindu worldviews and can have specific implications in the NICU. This is confirmed in the responses I received
to an anonymous online survey that I created and sent out to adults, living in
the United States, who self-identify as Hindu. To unpack the six characteristics
discussed earlier, listen to the voices of those who responded to the survey.

Though seventy-eight individuals completed portions of the survey, twenty-
seven answered one or more of the specific questions regarding their religious
beliefs as they relate to the care of a NICU patient. When asked to select a category
identifying their occupation, of the seventy-eight respondents, twenty-eight indicated "Healthcare Practitioner," ten indicated "Education" (e.g., K-12, college),
two indicated "Business, Financial or Management," and four indicated "Other"
(including one state government worker, one federal government worker, one
retired engineer, and one student). While nearly half of the respondents work
in the area of heath care, obviously their responses are not representative of all
Hindus working in health care. The survey itself is in no way a comprehensive

representation of Hindu perspectives. However, the responses provide us with insights into how some Hindus, living in the United States, respond to questions regarding their concerns when considering the care of a high-risk infant in the NICU. Following demographic questions, the first question on the survey was: "What would you identify as some challenges regarding the care of a high-risk newborn infant requiring NICU care?" Not surprisingly, we find a range in responses; here are a few examples:

- "Deciding end points to care."
- "End-of-life care issues."
- "Being able to identify the status or concerns of the family."
- "Lack of knowledge, emotional stress, health of baby, monetary worries, trusting medical staff."
- "Lack of maternal contact, sound communication between patient and medical care group."
- "Life or death."
- "Quality of life, potentially disability from illness and treatment, pain & suffering."
- "Anxiety involved for the parents and extended family; also, the cost, depending on the family's insurance of financial status."
- "The methods you take to keep the infant alive. How much are the infants suffering while we try to prolong their lives?"

The life expectancy and suffering of the infant are the biggest challenges that respondents identify. Among the responses, the type of medical care and technology and their application are the next highest concern, followed by interaction with and trust of the healthcare team taking care of the NICU infant.[21] These responses are probably shared by most, if not all, families, regardless of religious commitments. This reiterates the need for healthcare professionals to listen carefully to what each individual family says about their challenges and needs.

When asked, "What are some religious beliefs that come to mind regarding the above situation [challenges faced in the NICU]?" again the answers varied:

- "None."
- "Belief in karma, reincarnation."
- "Karma, dharma, reincarnation."
- "Child's karma, family's suffering, and the balance of the horoscopes."
- "Not too many—I would be aggressive in using the best medical technology has to offer in helping to save the neonates."
- "I believe truth is the ultimate dharma of a person, especially a caregiver."

• "Making sure there are no beef products in feedings ... pooja's [Hindu form of worship/prayer][22] in NICU, such as Chhati Pooja."

In these responses alone, we see two of the six characteristics explicitly named and the four others implied, along with the mention of a few specific cultural and ritual practices.

First, it is no surprise that there is a great deal of diversity in the responses to all the questions. While this is true for all religious traditions, the multivalent nature of traditions within Hinduism highlights this diversity. The first, "None," response is an example of someone who, even though identifying as Hindu, does not see religion playing a role in this situation. For others, their Hindu faith influences concerns over the suffering of the infant to the ingredients in the feedings.

Some respondents express a desire for healthcare professionals to be sensitive to this diversity within Hinduism. Two responses to the question, "From your knowledge/experience of Hinduism: What would be important for neonatal caregivers (doctors, nurses, etc.) to know about Hindu beliefs and values ... ?" are as follows:

• "Understand the diversity of our faith, and cultural variances, with people from different parts of India, and of course consider the added influences of westernization, no one size fits all."
• "The beliefs and customs [of Hindus] may seem crude or primitive but in fact they are quite profound and important for the patients."

The first respondent wants healthcare professionals to be aware of the multiple ways in which Hinduism is embodied, and he or she does not want typologies or "recipes" applied. The second quotation reflects someone who fears, or may have experienced, someone disregarding his or her beliefs or considering them to be "crude" or "primitive." If we engage our patients or their families with an attitude of cultural humility, perhaps the importance of this person's beliefs would be heard, and we would be able to communicate this. In addition, in response to a question regarding what ritual practices might be relevant in caring for a NICU patient, a respondent said: "I do not know about ritual practices; however, I would hope the high-risk newborns are treated with respect and care and love." This, the desire to be treated with respect, care, and love, is a response probably shared by most, if not all. If we listen to each family, each member, and figure out what respect, care, and love looks like to them, then we can respond accordingly.

Returning to the responses to the question regarding what religious beliefs come to mind regarding NICU situations, we not only see the multivalent nature of Hindu tradition but also have explicit mention of the second and third characteristics of Hinduism, namely karma and dharma. While the meanings of karma and dharma were discussed previously, here is how a few individuals talk about them in their own words. Regarding karma: one respondent muses that some might feel they are "being tested for past sins," or that the "whole sense of karma, birth and rebirth, might give some strength." Another respondent writes,

- "In Hindu religion, we believe in past life karma influencing the present life. So parents can pray that the effect of their past karma may be reduced and help them see their infants get normal."

Yet another says,

- "What right do I have to prolong the infant's life and make him/her suffer, if this is how things are meant to be? Perhaps this is my lot, my destiny, the karma that we (the infant and I) are experiencing."

Finally, one explicitly indicates that the idea of karma brings comfort, writing,

- "I think that there would be a certain sense of peace (I hope), that if I have to withdraw care, that this is just one step in my child's eternal journey. Perhaps, having lived a short but pure and virtuous life, his return to this world in his next life would be met with much better fortune. I would take comfort that his/her soul would encounter a brighter future."

Through these quotations, we see examples of how karma is understood and how people see it functioning as they try to make sense of their NICU situation, whether as parents, family members, or healthcare providers.

Dharma also appears in many answers throughout the survey. When asked what beliefs come to mind, or what values play a role in determining what to do, many respondents mention dharma. As a family member, one respondent says that it is our "duty to alleviate pain and suffering and if possible, save a life—duty to do one's dharma rather than fall apart in despair."
A physician's response:

- "As a Hindu, I feel [that it] is my dharma to be a good doctor and provide best care possible to my patients."

Another health care provider says,

- "As a Hindu, I believe in using all that western medicine has to offer to save a high risk neonate. None of us can predict the long term outcome. It is just our duty/dharma to do our best to save a life."

When discussing the challenges faced in the NICU, one writes,

- "Just be truthful and allow karma and dharma to guide you."

These quotations reflect how dharma takes on multiple meanings, especially when one considers contexts. The physician has one dharma, duty, while a family/support person has another. An individual acts (karma) according to her dharma and, for many, this coincides with the idea of reincarnation.

The characteristic of the underlying unity of all life is the warp through which karma and dharma are woven related to the belief of reincarnation. As discussed previously, the soul is Brahman (essence of everything) and therefore eternal. This belief is reflected in a number of responses that also talk about reincarnation. Here are a few examples:

- "The value of rebirth and revival. Each soul born on this earth has a purpose and that when that purpose is over, the soul moves on. The body is but a vehicle for the soul. The soul (the atman) is forever. Dust unto dust is what the body is all about."
- "The understanding of atman, as eternal, suffering as part of karma."
- "I do not believe that death, is an end, it is part of the journey, that we have to go thru, a different act in a different scene in the future."
- "I do believe that life is precious, but I also believe that life is but a part of the journey that my soul experiences. As I get older I get more convinced that death signifies the beginning of another phase of my life and not its end."
- "Life does not end with death, the soul does go [on] and [is] reborn. So one should not worry too much if one person will die. If [the] future is a difficult life, avoid helping."
- "I would have to ask honestly which course would be best for the infant. If the cessation or withdrawal of treatment was the best course, in terms of preventing suffering, this would be accepted with sorrow, but also in the hope that this soul will continue on its journey to another rebirth, or to Liberation."
- "When an infant's medical condition, in spite of all our efforts, does not improve, it's time to let her/him go. Because it means that their purpose [dharma] has been fulfilled and they're ready to leave this earth. People may wonder what was that purpose. Perhaps it was just come to this earth as someone's child. We don't know. All we know is that that soul is ready to move on and we should let it go."

These quotations demonstrate that commitments to an underlying unity of all life, karma, and dharma ground a belief in reincarnation. Again, though there may be a shared commitment to a particular belief, what one actually does can be very different. When applied to infants diagnosed with Trisomy 13, Tay-Sachs disease, or Lesch-Nyhan syndrome or who are for other reasons in the NICU, some argue for doing everything possible to save their life, while others might be more willing to allow these infants to die. However, in all the responses, there is a sense that the end of this life is not the end of the journey of the soul itself. These beliefs, as one respondent says, "would give great strength. Not necessarily solace, but the tools to get through the traumatic situation."

Of the six characteristics presented at the beginning of this chapter, the centrality of society is indirectly present in the survey responses. First, discussions of dharma presume that one is talking about duty in the context of family and the larger community. Dharma is not a singular, individualistic notion; it is one's duty, one's role in society, order and law within a community, and so on. Second, a number of respondents presume a context of a larger community:

- "They [beliefs and values] would compel me to do whatever I could to ensure the best possible care for the infant; or, depending on my role [dharma], to support the family enduring this situation. We actually had something like this happen in our local Hindu community, and it was heartening to see how the entire community came together to support the family, bringing food to the home, helping look after the other children in the family, and so on."

When listing important elements to understand for Hindus, one writes,

- "The wide varieties of practices, and individual freedom, of each sect, and community, and role of elders in [the] decision-making process, and their guidance."

Emphasizing both the centrality of society and the multivalent nature of Hinduism, consider these two quotations:

- "Generally, Hindu families tend to be quite male-centered. Depending on just how traditional the family is, there may even be instances where the men (or even just the single head of household) will make all the decisions without consulting any women, including the mother of the child. Women may not even be allowed to be in the child's presence."

As opposed to:

- "The mother's role will likely be most central. She may require special counseling if she feels that what has happened to her baby is somehow due to her own bad karma or negligence. An alternative interpretation should be provided, such as that this is an opportunity to do seva."

Either way, in a male-centered family or community, or in one where a mother plays a central role, community is central. In addition, *seva* means service. Seva is an important component to a successful, vibrant community.

Ahimsa, the sixth Hindu characteristic, also appears in the responses. A few are:

- "I imagine values of nonharming, care, minimizing interventions that are not natural or likely to produce long-term effects or side-effects."
- "If the treatment is making the infant suffer unnecessarily, then the decision to strop treatment is valid."
- "Premature termination, excessive medication, harm to the infant and/or mother."
- "Treat the patient to the best of your ability but if at all possible limit suffering. Don't prolong life if the effort is futile."

In these responses, we see an explicit desire to do the least amount of harm. Physicians and other healthcare professionals are expected to do their very best; however, they are not to utilize technology just because it is available. The baby's experience and that of the family need to be in the forefront of concern. Treat the infant, all the while keeping an eye to causing the least amount of harm possible.

I have discussed six characteristics of Hindu thought and seen a variety of ways they come into play for people who self-identify as Hindu. As healthcare providers, you are probably still looking for particular practices, rituals, or the like that your Hindu patients and family may want to do. There were a number of responses to the question: "What ritual practices or considerations might be relevant for the treatment of a high-risk newborn infant?" Having the ability to pray, conduct a puja,[23] and recite mantras were the frequent replies. Last rites, naming ceremonies, visits from Hindu priests, and readings from particular religious texts were other practices discussed. One individual responded,

- "Not too familiar, but the recitation of certain mantras during his/her battle for recovery would certainly be welcome. Having a pundit come and perform a blessing or a puja would likely be something we would desire. In that realm, given how central fire is to the practice of Hindu rituals, this might cause conflict with staff and hospital officials where it's likely the lighting of a fire and/or burning of incense would be deemed impossible."

An open flame in a NICU is obviously not permissible; however, speaking with the family provides the opportunity to learn what they desire and together they, health care providers and family members, can find creative options that satisfy the desires of the family and rules of the hospital.[24] A number of respondents indicated they do not follow any particular rituals. So, again, remember that claiming a religious tradition is not an indicator of any particular practice: be ever mindful that nothing is monolithic. Emphasizing the need to assess the desires of each individual family, one respondent said: "Whatever that particular family believes in, you can't have a single recipe for ALL HINDUS."

I began this chapter with a discussion of cultural humility because it is a necessary frame of mind if one desires to be an excellent healthcare provider. Technical knowledge and skills are of course required; equally important is someone who has cultivated the skills of listening. The six characteristics of Hindu thought and the voices of Hindus living in the United States are presented with the goal of enabling NICU healthcare providers to listen more carefully to patients and families. Having an attitude of cultural humility enables healthcare providers to listen, learn, and not to label or categorize. Emphasizing this point, here are a couple of responses to the question: "What would be important for neonatal caregivers (doctors, nurses, etc.) to know about Hindu beliefs and values to be of the most assistance in this context?"

- "Mainly that we believe in reincarnation and therefore we may be a bit more willing to withdraw care or allow death than those of other faiths. They [healthcare professionals] would need to understand this so as to not judge those that might make these types of decisions that they themselves may not agree with."
- "That although we believe in the enduring soul and in rebirth, that family is extremely important to us and we would want to do all that is possible to ensure the best possible quality of life for the infant. That any decision to discontinue treatment is not made callously or out of a disregard for human life, as people ignorant of Hinduism might mistakenly think."
- "That Hindus care as much about infants in such situations as members of any other religious community, but also may tend to be more pragmatic if the situation requires that treatment be discontinued. This, again, is not callousness, but an acceptance that death is a natural part of life, and that rebirth is a certain reality."

Finally,

- "I am a spiritual person. . . . I think the problem with ICU care in general is that doctors tend to think 100% scientifically and organ based. How are the lungs doing? How are the kidneys doing? How is the heart doing? Sometimes they forget about the 'whole person' or being they are treating. I think prayer, energy, and family love make a huge difference in outcome."

As NICU healthcare providers move forward offering the highest of technical medical skills and technology available, remember you are indeed engaging a whole human being, a family, and indeed the entire process of Shiva's dance. The title of this chapter is "Shiva's Babies," because Shiva, the Lord of the Dance, creates, sustains, and destroys the world in his 108 dances. Those of you caring for the NICU infant, hold in your hands this entire process! While this chapter hopefully provided you with ideas and insights into some workings of Hindu worldviews, if you maintain an attitude of cultural humility, you are more likely to become aware of the particular worldviews of your patient's family. These insights can enable you to speak in ways that the family will better understand. These conversations can build trust and understanding, thereby enabling you to deliver the best care in the most effective manner.

Notes

1. Cynthia Foronda et al., "Cultural Humility: A Concept Analysis," *Journal of Transcultural Nursing* 27, no. 3 (2016): 212–13. In the authors' discussion of the consequences of cultural humility, they refer to a number of other studies that demonstrated positive outcomes, including "mutual empowerment, partnerships, respect, optimal care . . . building honest and trustworthy relationships . . . effective treatment . . . and improved care."
2. Melanie Tervalon and Jann Murray-Garcia, "Cultural Humility versus Cultural Competence: A Critical Distinction in Defining Physician Training Outcomes in Multicultural Education," *Journal of Health Care for the Poor and Underserved* 9, no. 2 (May 1998): 117–25.
3. Foronda et al., 210.
4. Ibid., 213.
5. For a discussion of how I identify these specific characters of Hindu thought, see: Swasti Bhattacharyya, *Magical Progeny, Modern Technology: A Hindu Bioethics of Assisted Reproductive Technology* (New York: State University of New York Press, 2006).
6. *Rg. Veda* 10:90.
7. *Mandaka Upanishad* 2.2.10–11.
8. *Atmabodha* 36–38.
9. *Laws of Manu*, 3.77–78.
10. It is also the stage of life where most grapple with issues such as we are discussing in this book: it is the time of life when people are getting married, having families, and building their careers.

11. S. Radhakrishnan, *The Hindu View of Life* (New Delhi: Indus, 1993), 76.
12. Sir Monier Monier-Williams, *Sanskrit-English Dictionary* (New York: Oxford University Press, 1995), 510.
13. *Bhagavad Gita*, 2.31–33.
14. Ibid., 2.50.
15. Radhakrishnan, 16.
16. *Bhagavad Gita* 3.35.
17. Radhakrishnan, 36.
18. *Bhagavad Gita* 3.5.
19. Katherine K. Young, "Hindu Bioethics," in *Religious Methods and Resources in Bioethics*, ed. Paul F. Camenisch (Boston: Kluwer Academic, 1994), 12.
20. M. K. Gandhi, *The Gospel of Selfless Action or The Gita According to Gandhi* (Ahmedabad: Navajavan Publishing House, 1946), 206.
21. Of the twenty-five individuals who wrote answers for this question, thirteen mentioned the suffering, life expectancy, or possible death of the infant. Two mentioned financial concerns.
22. The Smithsonian Institute provides an informative definition of puja and the elements it comprises. See https://www.asia.si.edu/pujaonline/puja/background.html (accessed May 2, 2017).
23. A puja is a ritual that often involves an oil lamp, incense, prayer (in the form of chants), and an offering (often food).
24. Getting to know the desires of the family and talking with them at appropriate times can be helpful in figuring out creative ways to incorporate traditional rituals. For example, in India, cremation is common. Traditionally, when a parent dies, the eldest son lights the funeral pyre. When my father died in the United States, I asked about the possibilities of allowing my brother, the eldest son, to push the button that ignited the incinerator. I had no idea if it was even permissible for us to be in the room. They accommodated us: the immediate family and priest conducted a brief ritual, and we were able to preserve the ancient tradition in a new way.

8

Life Before Birth

Buddhist Perspectives on Neonatal Care

Karma Lekshe Tsomo

The field of applied Buddhist ethics is evolving in a rich intellectual and technological climate that is both exhilarating and terrifying. Current debates about biomedical issues stretch Buddhist thinking beyond traditional philosophical boundaries and challenge the perceived boundaries between religion and science. They also challenge traditional thinking about what it means to be a human being and conventional understandings of what constitutes knowledge and wisdom. These debates expand the conversation about the beginnings of life to include questions about practical decisions for which no definitive scriptural guidelines exist. The questions are not simple, and the answers are still tentatively unfolding, complicated by the intriguing religious diversity of contemporary society. Multi-religious families are now challenged by bioethical decisions that require deeper understandings of both science and the tenets of traditional faiths as well as new spiritual traditions.

This chapter considers ethical issues related to the care of high-risk newborns, including questions about the cessation or withdrawal of treatment, within the context of Buddhist ethical values and principles.[1] A key point for reflection is the ontological and moral status of the premature or newborn infant from a cross-cultural Buddhist perspective. The objective is to explore the diversity of Buddhist beliefs and practices related to the care of newborns with congenital health challenges and decision making by religious leaders, medical professionals, legal experts, and parents.

Questions of ethical decision making are approached very differently among the widely diverse Buddhist traditions that have developed over 2,500 years. The world's Buddhists belong to divergent philosophical schools and practice traditions, many of which are influenced by non-Buddhist beliefs and practices. These philosophical and practice traditions developed over many centuries and span vast cultural and geographical differences. Buddhists represent many diverse schools of thought, and their ideas are shaped by cultural values and indigenous beliefs and practices that have nothing to do with Buddhism. To complicate matters, Buddhists acknowledge no central institutional authority, such as the Vatican, that is entrusted to make decisions for the Buddhist tradition overall. Buddhist clerics are often consulted about medical decision making, but they do not speak with one voice, and they may not feel confident to give well-informed advice about the issues.

The Buddha lived in India during the fifth or sixth century B.C.E. Buddhists today in countries throughout the world live in very different cultural, political, and social settings and circumstances. We have no way to know how people at the time of the Buddha made decisions about the care of newborn infants, but we can be sure that they did not have the medical knowledge and advanced treatments that now exist and are available to at least the privileged among us today. The most fundamental principles that have guided Buddhist ethical decision making are to avoid taking life, to treat all sentient beings with compassion, and to culti-vate wisdom. The Buddha taught the law of cause and effect, or actions (*karma*) and their consequences. Through stories and examples, he explained how whole-some actions give rise to fortunate circumstances, whereas unwholesome actions result in unfortunate circumstances, either in this lifetime or future lives, placing special emphasis on the intention that motivates the action.

While these concepts are fairly straightforward, analogous to "As ye sow, so shall ye reap," we can only speculate about Buddhist responses to the many new ethical dilemmas that now confront humankind, extrapolating from what we can glean from the scriptures as they relate to infants and medical treatment. An age-old medical analogy refers to the sufferings of the human condition as the malady, the Buddha as the physician who diagnoses the malady, the Buddha's teachings as the medicine that can remedy the malady, and the monastic com-munity as the nurses who help suffering beings by administering the medicine.

In one scriptural passage, we learn that the Buddha admonished a group of monks for not taking care of a fellow monk who was sick with dysentery.[2] He said, "Monks, you have no mother, you have no father, who might tend to you. If you don't tend to one another, who then will tend to you? Whoever would tend to me, should tend to the sick." In the story, he describes the characteristics of patients who are easy to tend to and patients who are difficult to tend to. He describes the characteristics of nurses who are fit to tend to the sick and those who are not. In some texts, such as Ghosaka's *Abhidharmamāmrtaśāstra*, sick persons are included in the list of those who are "fields of merit," that is, worthy objects of generosity.[3] Nowhere, however, as far as I know, does he discuss care for newborns or sick children.

There are stories about women suffering the loss of their children that may give us some clues, however.[4] One is a famous story about a pregnant woman named Patacara, whose husband dies from a poisonous snakebite while chop-ping wood to shelter her during a storm. After the trauma of losing her husband

and both her children, she returns home to find that her mother, father, and brother all died during the storm and are burning on a funeral pyre. Through the experience of these traumas, she realizes the truth of suffering so deeply that she achieves "the deathless state," *nirvana*—liberation from attachment and the suffering it causes. She goes on to become a master of monastic discipline. The text begins by reminding the reader of the sufferings of women:

Stressful, painful, is the woman's state:
so says the tamer of tamable people.
Being a co-wife is painful.
Some, on giving birth once,
slit their throats.
Others, of delicate constitution,
take poison.
In the midst of a breech-birth
both [mother and child] suffer destruction.[5]

Another famous story tells of a woman named Kisagotami who is heartbroken because of the loss of her only child. After she becomes deranged with grief, she approaches the Buddha, who promises to restore her dead child if she can find a sesame seed from a home where there has never been a death. Delighted by his promise, she goes from door to door, but finding no home where no one has died, she realizes the truth of death and impermanence. She sings a verse extolling the benefits of conquering grief and sorrow through her realization of death's universality. These stories are familiar to most Buddhists, as they are told over and over again and also presented in popular drama performances. The lesson taught through these stories—that death is inevitable—helps human beings recognize that the pain of loss they experience at the death of a loved one derives from attachment. The greater attachment one has to a loved one, the greater pain one experiences at the time of their loss. Therefore, recognizing that death is a natural part of the life cycle helps Buddhists to deal with the grief they feel when they lose a loved one. This is not to say that ordinary Buddhists do not suffer when their friends and family members die; they do. This also does not imply that a deep experience of suffering is absolutely necessary for spiritual realization, but personal suffering often serves as a catalyst for awakening. Even for ordinary families, understanding the inevitability of suffering and death helps parents and siblings to accept the loss of a child more easily. Being able to relinquish their clinging and attachment enables them to let go of their sorrow at separation more quickly. In the case of a seriously disabled or high-risk child, being able to recognize one's attachment and relinquish their bond to the child may enable the parents to more easily recognize when extraordinary medical treatment is futile.

Buddhists would not want to cause harm to a child or an adult either physically or emotionally. Both in theory and practice, all beings should be treated with compassion, regardless of their age—newly born, mature, or elderly. When faced with a dilemma that requires balancing benefit and harm, most Buddhists would endeavor to practice compassion for the child. Most would stop short of taking the life of a child, even a severely disabled one. Most would do everything they could to care for the child, to the best of their ability, but would not feel obligated to use extraordinary means to extend the life of a severely disabled child who is suffering greatly.

Another story indicates that care should be taken to avoid causing a woman to miscarry:

> Kālodāyin was a disciple whose skin was very black. He used to beg for food at night. A pregnant woman miscarried when she saw him in a flash of lightening in the dark of night. Then the Buddha stipulated that no one should beg for food after noontime.[6] In another version of the story, with no mention of skin color, the incident occurs at dusk, and the woman is startled by the figure of a monk going for alms as he rounds the corner of a house, causing her to miscarry. When the incident is reported to the Buddha, he sets forth a rule that prohibits monks from taking "untimely food," effectively requiring them to fast for eighteen hours a day, out of concern for the lives of unborn fetuses.

Stories such as these highlight four fundamental principles that help guide Buddhist ethical decision making: nonharm, loving kindness, compassion, and wisdom. These principles shape attitudes toward all sentient beings, that is, all beings who possess consciousness, including animals. These four principles are not simply theoretical, but rather are intended to apply to everyday life situations. These principles apply to healthcare decisions for the sick newborn and all other situations.[7] Many texts emphasize the importance of balancing wisdom and compassion. In the case of a severe and terminal disability, most Buddhists would find it difficult to justify aggressive treatment, but would ordinarily care for the infant with love until the end of his or her life. In such a case, most Buddhists would not condemn parents who made a decision to withhold or withdraw treatment. The same attitude and care that are given to the high-risk newborn would also be extended to older pediatric or adult patients. All are equally sentient beings and equally have the potential to achieve liberation.

At the time of the Buddha, most people in India lived in subsistence economic circumstances and relied on natural herbs to treat various illnesses and health conditions. Without a way to extend their lifetimes artificially, they died of natural causes. Hundreds of millions of people still do so today. They often rely on the guidance of religious specialists such as Buddhist monks (and sometimes nuns) when faced with a decision about health care, especially if the condition is serious. In addition, in some communities, it is not uncommon for Buddhists to consult indigenous healers to guide their medical decision making. In some Buddhist cultures, mediums may also be consulted. Many Buddhist societies acknowledge the presence of invisible beings, gods, and spirits whose existence is factored into the Buddhist equation in thinking about healthcare and medical decision making. Among younger people who have received a Western education, reliance on divination and spirit mediums seems to be on the decline, but as they get older and begin to face more difficult decisions, they may also seek out these channels of information, like their parents. This conciliatory view is evident in the advice His Holiness the Dalai Lama gives to Tibetans, "Do the rituals *and* take the medicine."

While living in Tibetan society for fifteen years, on several occasions I consulted or served as a translator in interactions with Buddhist *lamas* (spiritual teachers) who were famed for their record of "accurate" divinations. The majority of questions posed to these *lamas* are health related. The *lama* is considered a pure channel for information from specific deities. All recommendations and decisions are for the express purpose of avoiding suffering and the various kinds of unwholesome actions that will lead to suffering, based on the law of cause and effect. The duty of parents to care for their children is widely assumed, and the importance of sparing children from suffering goes unquestioned. Not all treatments are medical. Some ailments may be treated with rituals to dispel negative interferences or "harmers" (*no ba*); others may be addressed with religious practices such as saving the lives of animals, which are intended to accumulate good karma to offset whatever unwholesome karma from the past may be causing the ailment. Even though the practice is discouraged from an orthodox perspective, in some Buddhist societies, spirit mediums may be consulted for remedies, and some are specially renowned for their efficacious divinations for children.[8] In Tibetan cultural areas, *lamas* are often consulted in weighing which medical options will be most efficacious, both in the short term and in the long run, and the best time for performing funerals and cremations.

One case I know of illustrates a clash of cultural mores related to healthcare decision making.[9] While I was living in Dharamsala, India, a child was born with encephalitis. The parents were understandably upset and, as is customary, decided to seek the advice of a religious specialist to determine the best course of treatment. The options generally include Tibetan, Ayurvedic, or Western medical systems. The *lama* who was consulted counseled against seeking medical treatment at a Western hospital. Under pressure from a Canadian woman, the parents finally decided to seek Western medical treatment for the child. I have no information about the course of treatment prescribed, but I know that the child lived for three years in great pain, causing immense suffering to the child, the parents, and other loved ones and friends in the community. In the aftermath, the Canadian woman doubted the wisdom of her decision in insisting that the parents take the child to a Western hospital for treatment rather than letting nature take its course. She felt great remorse and worried for years afterward that, unable to bear the early death of the child, she had inadvertently caused tremendous suffering and confusion.

Some Buddhist texts portray the notion of birth in problematic terms. Owing to ignorance and delusion, beings create unwholesome actions that result in birth, sickness, old age, and death. On one hand, a birth is to be celebrated because to take birth in a human body is an unparalleled opportunity for spiritual evolution and liberation. On the other hand, a birth is sad because to take birth necessarily entails many problems, frustrations, and physical and emotional pain. Birth inevitably ends in death and, unless one achieves liberation in that lifetime, further rebirth. Birth inevitably leads to death and is, therefore, an unsatisfactory experience. Life is believed to begin at conception, and gestation is described as nine or ten months long. The texts vividly portray the sufferings of the fetus, who is said to experience pain when the mother eats or drinks hot or cold food or beverages, moves abruptly, jumps, has sex, and so on. The texts also vividly portray the sufferings of the newborn, who is said to experience the pain of being born like being squeezed between two mountains. Under the circumstances, the gentle reception of the new arrival is of utmost importance. The infant should be handled with great care, wrapped in soft cloth, and protected from all harm.

An indication of the ontological and moral status of the newborn can be seen in *mizuko kuyo*. This is a ritual (*kuyo*) performed in Japan for "water babies" (*mizuko*), referring to fetuses, newborns, stillborn babies, and young children who die prematurely. The ritual, performed at a temple, is thought to be efficacious in relieving the pain of the being whose life has ended so early, whether through abortion, miscarriage, illness, or accident. The intention is to help the *mizuko* to attain a favorable rebirth. It is also performed to assuage the psychological pain of the parents. There are also those who request the ritual to ward off any negative effects from the wandering spirit of the *mizuko*.[10] Temples receive donations or may charge a fee for performing the ritual. As a result, in recent years, a large number of temples with dubious pedigrees have sprung up. Some temples that perform the ritual are run like businesses. These temples and the practice of *mizuko kuyo* generally have come under criticism that they take advantage of those who have lost children for material gain. The practice of *mizuko kuyo* has also been introduced in some American Buddhist communities, where it is regarded as a healthy method for dealing with emotional pain and conflicts that might be experienced at the loss of a child, especially through abortion.

All phenomena arise from causes, and the human body is typically used as an example. A human rebirth is regarded as the result of good moral conduct, a prosperous rebirth is the result of generosity, and fortunate physical characteristics are the result of specific wholesome actions. For example, those who speak gently in one lifetime have beautiful voices in their next lifetime, those who are gentle and kind have beautiful features, and vice versa. The texts also explain that unpleasant physical characteristics are the result of unwholesome actions in past lives. Congenital anomalies, birth defects, neonatal illnesses, and similar misfortunes are commonly understood by ordinary people to be the result of the child's actions in a past life. It is important to understand the concept in the context of multiple rebirths and the theory of cause and effect. There is no sense that the child or the parents are being punished for their misdeeds because there is no entity that delivers punishments. Misfortunes are understood to be related to one's own actions, either in this life or some previous life, in a natural process related to actions and their consequences. Parents will often perform good deeds, such as making an offering to a temple or monastics, to accumulate merit that will offset any unwholesome actions created in the past, either by the parents or the child, in hopes of having a healthy child.

In Buddhist philosophy and Buddhist societies, newborns are considered sentient beings, that is, beings who possess consciousness and are capable of experiencing feelings: pleasant, painful, or neutral. Newborns, like other sentient beings, take birth repeatedly in a continuum of countless lifetimes over immense expanses of time. In these various lifetimes, they take birth in myriad different forms and myriad world systems, in a vast array of relationships, according to their karma. Their experiences of various degrees of fortune and misfortune are not caused or created by any higher power, but rather are regarded as the result of actions they have committed in past lifetimes, extending back to beginningless time. The realm of rebirth in which one is born—as a god, human being, animal, and so on—is the consequence of actions created in the past, whether wholesome, unwholesome, or neutral. Taking birth as a human being, for example, is regarded as the consequence of wholesome moral conduct; taking birth as an animal is the consequence of less admirable actions, for example, lazy or beast-like behavior. One's life circumstances—one's appearance, intelligence, predispositions, family circumstances, and so on—are also the result of one's actions in previous lives. Being born into a prosperous family is regarded as the consequence of the practice of generosity; being born poor is the result of stinginess. Being born with physical weaknesses or disabilities is regarded as the consequence of actions such as harming other sentient beings. Being born with a terminal illness may be the result of having harmed or cut short the life span of other sentient beings.

Ordinary Buddhists' views on life are influenced by their understanding of the law of cause and effect. The theory of cause and effect operates impersonally, like a natural process of the universe: actions and reactions, cause and effect. There is no prime mover or manipulator of the process of birth, death, and rebirth (*samsara*). There is no sense of blaming those who experience misfortunes; on the contrary, the teachings on cause and effect help Buddhists to develop understanding and empathy. There is no sense that those who suffer misfortunes are condemned to suffer; on the contrary, there are many practices for creating wholesome actions to offset or mitigate the effects of one's unwholesome actions. These wholesome actions include kindness, compassion, generosity, meditating, chanting the Buddha's teachings, and so on. It is important to note that these views are in no way intended as a condemnation of the infant or the parents. There is no sense in which the person who experiences misfortune is regarded as "getting what they deserve." Everyone has made mistakes and has an opportunity to do things differently in the future. Even a small action, such as giving a mouthful of food to a dog, is an opportunity to accumulate good karma and help ensure one's own future well-being.

As far as I know, there is no specific mention of premature babies in the Buddhist texts.

However, the suffering of a newborn with impaired faculties can be understood within the framework outlined previously. The parents of a medically challenged infant will typically feel sad, even distraught, but their understanding of the law of cause and effect helps them to put things in perspective. Their family is not the only one to experience misfortune; myriad other families are also experiencing similar sufferings. It is said that the tears each one of us has shed throughout our lifetimes are enough to fill the great oceans. The decisions that Buddhist parents make regarding palliative care for their newborn child will be guided by their ethical principles, such as compassion and nonharm. Because the infant has been born into their family, they will typically understand that they have a special karmic affinity with the child and, therefore, have a special responsibility to care for the child with love and compassion.[11]

Birth as a result of karmic affinity is mentioned in certain Buddhist texts that recount stories of beings who are born in the same family for many lifetimes. The decision to take birth in a particular circumstance is graphically portrayed in Tibetan paintings that picture the consciousness of a being taking conception during the moment of sexual union of a man and woman. Scenes depicting such a conception can be found in Tibetan medical texts on embryology. Accounts of Tibetan Buddhist women who have special dreams at conception and during pregnancy are common. Feeling a karmic connection with the being who has joined their family may create a special sense of connectedness and tenderness for the newborn child. The belief in karmic affinities through many lifetimes may cause the parents to feel an especially deep sorrow at the suffering of a severely ill or disabled child. At the same time, Buddhists acknowledge that the newborn has his or her own mental continuum with karmic imprints from the past. Further, Buddhists recognize that all sentient beings have been closely related to one another at some point since beginningless time, and we have all shed immeasurable tears at the loss of our children. Philosophically at least, Buddhists know that the identities of living beings shift from lifetime to lifetime and that clinging to and grasping at these illusory forms is foolish. Clearly, this knowledge does not erase the pain of giving birth to an infant who is suffering, but it may make it easier to accept. Recognizing their limited understanding of medical science, parents may feel overwhelmed with grief and uncertainty, but they will use whatever knowledge they have to make wise and compassionate decisions. They will also call on others whom they consider wise, such as Buddhist monastics, clerics, and others in the community who can speak knowledgeably about the Buddha's teachings in making medical decisions for the newborn.

For Buddhists, the question of how to care for the critically ill newborn or newborn of borderline viability is approached within the framework of balancing short-term and long-term harm and benefit to the child. Under the circumstances, the parents are in most cases necessarily dependent on the medical staff for advice regarding medical decisions, so establishing rapport and trust with parents is crucial. Buddhist clerics are not educated in the technologies or the moral issues involved in the intense atmosphere of the neonatal intensive care unit (NICU); many are not even especially well educated in Buddhist philosophy. In the case of irregular births, they will do their best when congregants call on them, but their knowledge and their capacity for empathy in unfamiliar situations such as the neonatal setting may be very limited. The parents will be most receptive to the advice of gentle, caring people and may become confused and upset if they feel that medical personnel are brusque, rude, or uncaring toward the infant. It is unquestioned that the parents have a duty to protect a critically ill child, especially a vulnerable newborn. Aggressive interventions with kindness may be acceptable for the long-term benefit of the infant, but rough handling, treatments that cause excessive suffering, and tests that cause harm without any understandable benefit to the newborn are to be avoided. A pure motivation on the part of all caregivers is assumed and expected. This is consistent with the Buddhist ethic of loving kindness and compassion. In the unfortunate case that parents have two sick infants, impartial loving kindness is all the more important. Gentle words and actions are healing, especially in relations with those who are ill, helpless, and vulnerable, such as newborns. Because the newborn is not able to make decisions and the parents must assume the major responsibility, they may feel especially sad and distraught. This is particularly true of first-generation immigrant Buddhists who may not be comfortable or confident with English interactions. Treating the parents with respect and gentleness is therefore very important.

The reason that the topic of life and death decision making for neonates is such an emotionally charged issue is precisely because of the vulnerable status of newborns and because there is no definitive answer to the ethical dilemmas surrounding their care. To this, the Buddhists add the immense value of achieving a human rebirth, with its rare potential to realize liberation. Taken together, these factors make the situation all the more charged. In earlier times, in cases of severe illness or disability and at the end of life, Buddhists would do all they could to provide medical treatment and nutrition to maintain life, make patients comfortable, and create merit on their behalf. Beyond that, they ordinarily let nature take its course. There is no obligation to artificially extend a person's lifetime because the methods used to extend life could cause the person more pain and additional health problems.

In premodern societies, end-of-life decisions were simpler to make because neonatal technologies and sophisticated treatment options were not available. Although that may sound a bit brutal to the modern ear, reminders that death comes to all living beings are commonly heard among followers of all Buddhist traditions, even today. Perhaps the simpler scenario of letting nature take its course, while not erasing the sting of death, created a peaceful environment of acceptance that made death and loss easier to accept. I was once taken by a group of about twenty nuns to the funeral of a kind young man who had been one of the workers at their monastery. Although he had died just that day, his parents were remarkably calm at the funeral, their grief no doubt assuaged to some extent by the obvious appreciation and ritual prayers of the nuns for their son. Although all of my evidence is anecdotal, and little, if any, statistical evidence exists, it is my conviction that death awareness, rather than avoidance, informs the attitudes of Buddhists in diverse cultures in the care and treatment of children with a definitely limited future and likely death in infancy. I gained some first-hand experience of this when my 86-year-old father was in intensive care in central Florida at the time of the Terri Schiavo case, and his Buddhist doctors voiced very different prognoses about his future prospects and healthcare alternatives than did his fundamentalist Christian nurses.

In Buddhist texts and lore, it is said that living beings come into the present lifetime with a given life span, depending on the actions they have committed in the past, whether life-giving and life-nurturing or life-depriving and life-harming. The extent of one's life span is thought to be the result of one's actions, but it may also be affected by other mitigating factors. Sometimes, harmful actions of killing that might otherwise result in a rebirth of hellish suffering may be mitigated through the practice of wholesome actions, such as saving the lives of sentient beings. Buddhists in some societies regularly buy and release fish and animals to save their lives. Even if one's actions were seriously unwholesome, it is possible that the consequences may be mitigated by generating sincere regret, and the sooner one generates remorse, the better. For example, even if a person has committed a seriously nonvirtuous action such as murdering a human being, but sincerely repents and regrets having committed the action, the consequences may be mitigated. Instead of an extended stay in a hellishly painful existence, for example, the consequences might instead be experienced as a difficult or premature birth with serious health concerns.

The ethics of applying extraordinary methods of treatment depends on the situation. There are no standard limits of treatment that can be applied to all situations because medical conditions, family relations, and economic circumstances are all varied and contingent. Moreover, pain is variable in extent and duration. Even when a person is experiencing emotional or physical pain, this does not necessarily mean that living out the person's allotted life span or extending life is futile. Some Buddhists believe that by experiencing the results of one's previous nonvirtuous actions, karma has been expiated. About twenty-five years ago, I was bitten by a viper and almost died as a consequence. The yearlong treatment was extremely painful, but many Buddhists believed that through that experience, I had exhausted huge amounts of negative karma from the past. Because I did not retaliate against the snake, those karmic cycles came to an end. However painful the circumstances, it is understood that the misfortune is at least partially the result of one's own actions, and after the results have been mitigated or experienced, the effects of those causes are exhausted, so that is the end of the cycle.

Care at the bedside of the sick is crucially important, and although physical contact is somewhat more rare in Asian Buddhist cultures than in others, a caring attitude of loving kindness and compassion is highly valued. It is believed that the consciousness of a person who has just died may still be present at the site of death for a period of up to forty-nine days. For an infant, the likelihood of the consciousness remaining for more than one day is quite small. During this time, until the consciousness has left the body, it is important that the body be handled with extreme care and with minimal intervention. Overt expressions of grief, commotion, or abrupt handling during the dying process are to be avoided because they may inadvertently disturb the consciousness in its transition to the next life. Therefore, it is recommended that mourners express their grief in private, out of the range of hearing, and instead generate thoughts of loving kindness toward the dying person, family, attendants, and all concerned. If it becomes apparent that the infant's death is unavoidable, it is good to suggest that Buddhist parents may wish to invite a monk or nun to recite prayers, a valued practice of expressing compassion and accumulating merit on behalf of the child. In some traditions, the parents may recite prayers or mantras themselves or invite loved ones, friends, or religious specialists to do so. A number of popular verses serve as reminders that impermanence is the nature of all compounded things and that death comes to us all:

All things are impermanent.
They arise and pass away.
Having arisen they come to an end.
Their coming to peace is bliss.[12]

Recalling the true nature of the human condition helps Buddhists to cope with the illness and loss of their loved ones. These practices have the benefit of calming the mind and are regarded as blessings, especially in cases that may be terminal. Compassionate care for the patient's loved ones and caregivers is equally important. In fact, overall, it is safe to say that there can never be too much compassion.

Notes

1. Studies on Buddhism and bioethics include Damien Keown, *Buddhist and Bioethics* (London: Palgrave Macmillan, 2001); and Karma Lekshe Tsomo, *Into the Jaws of Yama, Lord of Death: Buddhist, Bioethics, and Death* (Albany: State University of New York Press, 2006).
2. "Kucchivikara-vatthu: The Monk with Dysentery" (Mv 8.26.1–8), by Thanissaro Bhikkhu. Access to Insight (Legacy Edition), November 30, 2013. See http://www.accesstoinsight.org/tipitaka/vin/mv/mv.08.26.01–08.than.html. For another translation of Mahavagga 8.26.1–8, see I. B. Horner, *Book of the Discipline* (Vinaya Pitaka), volume 4 (London: Pali Text Society, 1949), 431–34.
3. Typically, it is *bhikkhus* and *bhikkhunis* (fully ordained monastics) who are regarded as fields of merit. The list mentioned here also includes one's father, one's mother, the elderly, and the sick.
4. "Kisagotami Theri" (Thig 10), translated from the Pali by Thanissaro Bhikkhu. Access to Insight (Legacy Edition), November 30, 2013. See http://www.accesstoinsight.org/tipitaka/kn/thig/thig.10.01.than.html.
5. Ibid.
6. Rulu, *Thinking of Amitābha Buddha* (Bloomington, IN: AuthorHouse, 2012), 273.
7. Buddhist approaches to care for the dying include Margaret Coberly, *Sacred Passage: How to Provide Fearless, Compassionate Care for the Dying* (Boston: Shambhala, 2002); Thich Nhat Hanh, *No Death, No Fear: Comforting Wisdom for Life* (Berkeley: Parallax Press, 2003); Judith L. Lief, *Making Friends with Death* (Boston: Shambhala, 2001); and Sogyal Rinpoche, *Living and Dying in Tibetan Buddhism* (New York: HarperCollins, 2002).

8. Karma Lekshe Tsomo, "The Buddha and the Spirit World: Healing Praxis in a Himalayan Monastery," in *Buddhist Women in a Global Multicultural Community*, ed. Karma Lekshe Tsomo (Kuala Lumpur: Sukhi Hotu Press, 2008), pp. 129–38; and Ivette M. Vargas-O'Bryan, "Demon Diseases and Tibetan Medicine: The Interface between Religion and Science," in *As Long as Space Endures: Essays on the Kalacakra Tantra*, ed. Edward A. Arnold (Ithaca, NY: Snow Lion Publications, 2009), 364–84.

9. This conflict between traditional cultural views and contemporary perspectives of medical science mirrors, to some extent, the events recounted in Anne Fadiman, *The Spirit Catches You and You Fall Down: A Hmong Child, Her American Doctors, and the Collision of Two Cultures* (New York: Farrar, Straus and Giroux, 2012).

10. For a full discussion of these beliefs and practices (and their critics), see Helen Hardacre, *Marketing the Menacing Fetus in Japan* (Berkeley: University of California Press, 1999); William R. LaFleur, *Liquid Life: Abortion and Buddhism in Japan* (Princeton, NJ: Princeton University Press, 1994); Bardwell Smith, "Buddhism and Abortion in Contemporary Japan: Mizuko Kuyō and the Confrontation with Death," *Japanese Journal of Religious Studies* 15, no. 1 (1988): 3–24; and Dennis Klass and Amy Olwen Heath, "Grief and Abortion: Mizuko Kuyo, The Japanese Ritual Resolution," *Omega Journal of Death and Dying* 34, no. 1 (1996/1997): 1–14. For American perspectives on the practice, see Jeff Wilson, *Mourning the Unborn Dead: A Buddhist Ritual Comes to America* (New York: Oxford University Press, 2009).

11. See http://new.exoticindiaart.com/product/paintings/human-embryology-TT60.

12. Gil Fondsdal, "A Theravada Approach to Spiritual Care of the Dying and Deceased," in *Awake at the Bedside: Contemplative Teachings on Palliative and End-of-Life Care*, ed. Koshin Paley Ellison and Matt Weingast (Somerville, MA: Wisdom Publications, 2016), 170.

9

How Age-Old Cultural Tenets Complicate the Care of Premature or Sick Navajo Newborns

Maureen Trudelle Schwarz

At the time when I got into some problems with my pregnancy, . . . I was 36, and I was a very busy person. I worked; I had a job that was very stressful, too. I was taking classes. I was trying to carry my pregnancy as healthy as I could. One night I was coming back through where you were driving. . . . I turned to my turnoff and I accelerated to come in, just as I accelerated I hit a horse. So, that is what brought on all these complications. . . . The horse fell into the windshield and the head of it hit me right across my chest area. And I was, it was totally dark there was no light. . . . So, I walked back in the dark. My husband didn't know. There is no traffic here, nobody here.

—Mrs. J., Navajo Reservation, 7/3/05[1]

I was asked to contribute a chapter to this collection on American Indian religious teachings about the newborn as these are relevant to clinicians' and parents' medical decision making and care for premature and sick neonates. This area of investigation certainly holds rich material for reflection. The request is complicated, however, by the fact that there are currently 567 federally recognized sovereign Native American Nations, with 200-plus additional communities seeking such recognition. Each group has its own philosophical beliefs about the body, personhood, health, and illness, which directly influence individual wishes regarding care and treatment of premature and sick newborns. Thus, it would be impossible for any one person to speak for all indigenous groups in Native North America.

Having done ethnographic research among them since 1991, I can, however, provide some insight into how members of the *Diné* Nation (Diné is the preferred term of reference for the Navajo people, a term that translates in the native language to "The People") think about these issues. The Navajo are the largest federally recognized tribe, with a population of 330,000 people who call *Diné Bikéyah* (literally Navajoland) home, a vast expanse of land that extends over 27,000 square miles into Utah, Arizona, and New Mexico. As this chapter will demonstrate, contemporary Navajo people re-inscribe difference onto their bodies in the medical context to reiterate their Navajoness and distinguish it from non-Navajoness.

When a Navajo child is born prematurely in a reservation hospital, with serious health problems or birth defects, it will be taken by ambulance or helicopter to the nearest available neonatal intensive care unit (NICU), usually in Phoenix, Arizona, or Albuquerque, New Mexico, as was the case in Mrs. J. son's situation, because none of the hospitals on Navajo land have such facilities. As a result, parents of Navajo infants in NICUs and their supporting family members are out of their comfort zones when at a NICU with an ill child. This adds to their stress. They are extremely concerned about the child's condition, its causes and possible treatments, and the child's prognosis. Differences of opinion will invariably exist between the biomedical practitioners' and the Navajo family members' understandings of the causes, treatments, and appropriate care for the child.

Moreover, internationally mandated guidelines exist for the care and treatment of all sick children. The United Nations Convention on the Rights of the Child (CRC) was developed in 1989 to enumerate entitlements and protections to be afforded to every child in the world. The convention established the ultimate responsibility of all governments, institutions, and families to ensure that the rights of children are respected and that all actions dealing with children are performed in their best interest. The foremost CRC guideline to be followed in every NICU is "respecting the autonomy of the parents." Other major concerns are to "consider the best interests of the infant" and to respect "parents' values, culture, and religion."[2] Adhering to these guidelines requires taking the cultural beliefs and practices of the parents into consideration as an appropriate treatment plan is developed and implemented.

Despite the good intentions of these CRC guidelines, cultural clashes often occur because the morals and ethics of the families of infants and the ethics that medical personnel are trained to uphold differ. Several factors will be at play, for example, from the Navajo side when an infant is brought into an off-reservation NICU. Most important among them are those that make up the primary context of contemporary Navajo life: differences acknowledged between Navajo and non-Navajo; notions of contamination; and medical and religious pluralism. Additionally, numerous age-old Navajo tenets on the body and personhood are in play as parents and family members grapple with a child needing care in a NICU. These include but are not limited to relational notions of personhood; beliefs about how detached body parts retain lifelong influence; assumptions regarding the malleability of a newborn's body at birth; sound reasons against cardiopulmonary resuscitation (CPR) and blood transfusions; and convictions about the power of language. These are compelling forces that factor into what types of treatment will or will not be acceptable to the child's parents.

That such differences exist between the Navajo and allopathic providers is not unique. Understandings of the body, personhood, wellness, illness, and disability have consistently been important signifiers of difference between white colonizers and indigenous people around the globe—especially in the areas of hygiene and values.[3] This is true in Native North America as well as in other colonized countries.

In her full narrative, the Navajo mother who is referred to here as Mrs. J. touches on several of the key issues of concern to a contemporary Navajo woman caught in an unexpected situation that resulted in her newborn requiring the care of NICU staff. These concerns are best understood within the broader frame of traditional Navajo cultural tenets about health and illness. The narratives of Mrs. J. and other consultants reveal that contemporary Navajo therapeutic choices and practices are informed by a mix of moral beliefs deriving from a variety of perspectives—both ancient and contemporary.

When the Navajo were first colonized and incorporated into the United States' hierarchical system, attempts were made to exert dominance over what were at the time considered to be subordinate medical and religious systems in an intentional effort to replace them with what were deemed to be the preeminent systems—that is, the aim was for allopathic medicine and Christianity to dominate and replace the indigenous systems. This is no longer the case. At this point in time, the Indian Health Service seeks collaborative relationships between biomedicine and traditional Navajo healthcare choices. In terms of the lived experience of contemporary Navajo people, a noncompetitive model currently exists among allopathic medicine, traditional Navajo curing techniques, the Native American Church (NAC, which is a pan-Indian, semi-Christian, nativistic, redemptive religion focused on the ritual ingestion of peyote, with a long history), and most Christian forms of healing.[4] Competition does exist, however, between the previously mentioned curing systems and some Christian sects—for example, most Evangelical groups, which are exclusionary because of their own individual internal doctrines.

Countless Navajo people take advantage of biomedical technologies made available to them through the Indian Health Service or private medical care, without giving up their fundamental beliefs about health, illness, or curing.[5] None of the Navajo people with whom I consulted limit themselves to the use of one component of this pluralistic health system, such as traditional Navajo diagnosticians, herbalists, ceremonial practitioners, NAC practitioners, Christian pastors and congregations, or the care provided at Indian Health Service hospitals and clinics.

Concomitantly, the narratives contained in what are referred to as the oral histories—accounting for how the Navajo world came into being—remain extremely significant to many Navajo people; however, in the contemporary world, they no longer stand collectively as the only set of ancient stories or texts looked to for guidance. Thousands of Navajo people today celebrate spirituality through membership in introduced religions such as the various sects of Christianity or the NAC currently flourishing across the reservation. As a result, the Bible contains the historical chronicle to which thousands of Navajo families—now devout Christians from a variety of denominations—turn for counsel in today's world, while Navajo narratives of the healing powers of peyote experienced during NAC meetings are the explanations to which additional Navajo look. Moreover, Navajo accounts of miraculous recoveries through the laying on of hands or prayer circles serve as vivid examples of a contemporary genre of inspirational curing anecdotes centered on the power of Christian prayer.

With this profusion of healing beliefs and techniques available in the contemporary world, the majority of Navajo consulted report drawing on two or more of these sources in times of need. Moreover, regardless of what belief system or denomination any individual may claim, in the Navajo world, healing is a family affair, so traditional belief is almost always involved as an underlying frame that must be taken into consideration. This is the context in which decisions are made about how to care for family members when health problems such as premature birth, birth defects, or illness of an infant occur.

Navajo Philosophical Precepts

Traditional Navajo beliefs maintain that the universe preceded human existence. Thus, to understand the structural principles of Navajo philosophical orientation and the concerns raised by Mrs. J., it is necessary to first consider Navajo views of the cosmos and their place in it. Their oral histories take us deep into the womb of the earth, back to the beginning, to the first underworld, for, by Navajo accounts, the story of their origin contains the essence of all that exists or is ever possible.

It is paramount to point out that although these narratives detail the way every aspect of Navajo sacred geography was established, they are not now, nor have they ever been, considered *a religion*. Rather, they are understood to collectively form a charter given to the Navajo by the *Diyin Dine'é*, or "Holy People"; that is, they are considered to offer insight into *a way of life*. This was emphasized by many Navajo consultants.

In all the several hundred versions of the Navajo origin story transcribed to date, each subterranean world is referred to by color, with a progression from dark to light. Most accounts have three or four worlds: black, blue, yellow, and white.[6] Each underworld is portrayed as being in some state of chaos and disorder, resulting in the need for travel into the next world. The journey upward culminates in the emergence onto the earth's surface at the place of emergence.[7]

There, two of the Holy People, First Man and First Woman, built a sweat house in which *to think and sing the Navajo universe into existence*. They created a mountain for each of the four cardinal directions to denote Navajo sacred geography. The Navajo, who are known as the Earth Surface People, were created by "Changing Woman," who directed them to live within the geographical area demarcated by their four sacred mountains.[8] It was at this point that Changing Woman gave the Earth Surface People a charter, which provides information on how to live properly within their proscribed landscape. At this point, the newly created world is said to have been in a state of "natural order" or harmony, in which all living things were in their prescribed places and in their proper relationships with all other living things.

Navajo people traditionally classify illness by cause rather than symptoms—that is, diseases are not known by the symptoms they produce or by the parts of the body they affect; rather, a single cause may produce several different symptoms, and conversely, a single symptom may be caused by any of several agents. What is consistent is that Navajo believe that all illness is a result of disharmony, manifesting symptoms in the body and mind. The causes may be due to (1) violating a taboo, (2) doing or saying harmful things to people or other living things, (3) absorbing the aftereffects of an environmental event such as being near a tree when it is struck by lightning, or (4) as Mr. D. explains in the next section, being contaminated by exposure to an enemy or the harmful effects of witchcraft.

Contamination

MR. D.: In Navajo belief, any time that a foreigner cuts a body it needs to be corrected. And so Navajo, we believe that we should not be uh, cut, or any kind of lacerations or operations or any kind of surgical procedures done to a Navajo body—

M. S.: Any kind?

MR. D: Any kind. . . . That would be considered a, uh, contamination with a foreigner.

M. S.: What if it was a Navajo surgeon that did the surgery?
MR. D.: Navajo surgeon that would have done the surgery, that would be different.
M. S.: Oh?
MR. D.: They would not follow-up with a, an Enemy Way ceremony.[9]

As Edward Said noted in *Orientalism*, to some degree all societies derive a sense of identity negatively. This is most often accomplished by simply establishing a familiar space as "ours" and designating that beyond it as "theirs," without animosity.[10] When strangers enter your world with the intent to conquer it, however, a group is forced to make such a differentiation. By these means, people everywhere essentialize "others"—that is, diminish an entire society to a mass of soulless, unfeeling enemies; in the Navajo case, contact with their others became markedly dangerous because of possible *contamination*. Navajo cultural tenets regarding the potential danger of contamination from contact with a *bilaganna*, or a "Five-Fingered White Person," commonly referred to as an "Anglo" (that is, Euro-American—colonizer, in the American Southwest), with or without death being an element of the context, is of great relevance to parents making decisions about the care of their newborns in NICUs because they result in strong aversions to intimate contact with non-Navajo through CPR, blood transfusion, or, as noted previously by Mr. D., surgery.

Bilaganna are not the only enemies in the Navajo world. When I spoke with Dr. A., one of the few Navajo biomedical physicians working on the reservation, she delineated several other types of enemies recognized in the Navajo world. She notes, "White people have been considered the enemy ever since we were at war with white people and, uh, Mexican people, the Spanish are also the enemies. So, *anyone that has made war with the Navajo—those are all the enemies*."[11] If contamination results from any of these forms of contact, then only the *Enemy Way* (an elaborate nine-day ceremony seasonally restricted to summer) will help.[12]

As this demonstrates, health, illness, and healing are not neutral in the Navajo world. The source to which people attribute each of these phenomena offers important clues into how they see the contemporary moral and political landscape. Cultural memories of the first encounters between Navajo and Europeans establish paradigms for representations of "the contact," colonialism, and relationships with descendants of the colonizers or, in contemporary parlance: enemies. This is evident in Navajo narratives about illness and biomedical technologies. Physiological differences in Navajo bodies are recognized, marked, and retained in the contemporary medical context as a means by which to reaffirm Navajo collective identity and non-Navajo difference.

Analysis of Navajo oral history and contemporary narratives secured through ethnographic interviews reveals views on contamination by contact with non-Navajo as a lynchpin to understanding how medical discourse is an idiom through which Navajo people simultaneously express resistance to colonization and notions about collective identity. As a result, Navajo beliefs about contamination caused by contact with outsiders are of special importance to this case study. For example, the commentaries of those with whom I consulted on blood transfusion indicate that Navajo people divide human blood into the categories of Navajo and non-Navajo. And Navajo people are reluctant to allow the blood of a non-Navajo to be put into their bodies owing to concerns about contamination. Such concern applies to other biomedical procedures as well. In fact, there is a long history of overall avoidance of biomedicine on the part of Navajo people.

Although the Navajo signed a treaty with the American government in 1868, the first biomedical hospital was not established on the Navajo reservation until 1897 by the Protestant Episcopal Church. Many more followed. In the preantibiotics period of medicine, Navajo justifiably considered hospitals places of the dead to be avoided at all costs unless one was ready to expire.[13] Yet, a gradual shift toward hospital births began in the 1930s.[14] The actual time frame varied from area to area, depending on when individual hospitals and clinics were built on or near the Navajo reservation, on road conditions, and on a family's physical proximity to a hospital or clinic.[15] This shift gained momentum in the 1950s in response to several dramatic changes in the Navajo world, including increased school attendance and pressure from professionals for hospital births.[16] By the mid-1980s, 99% of all Navajo deliveries occurred in hospitals.[17]

Whether it is comfortable to accept or not, it is imperative to note that the United States remains a colonial society.[18] Like other Native Americans, Navajo people did not face a single catastrophic period with the arrival of Europeans. Rather, since their release from internment at Fort Sumner in 1868 and the establishment of a reservation for them at that time, the Navajo have been in a relationship of constant domination and control by the larger American society. Colonial assault has been repeatedly demonstrated through repression of their native language and traditions, threats to Navajo land and resources, and impediments to the freedom to live according to the teachings of the Holy People. These concerns, coupled with social and health problems including economic underdevelopment and chronic unemployment, problems associated with alcohol, and high rates of diabetes and illnesses associated with improperly regulated mining, have resulted in historical trauma. It is within this context of rapid cultural change and fragmentation that Navajo people have gradually searched out new sources of curing powers, including those available from Christianity, the NAC, and biomedical technologies.

Challenges of Medical and Religious Plurality

The challenges of navigating religious and medical pluralism through times of family illness are beautifully illustrated by a story told by Mr. W. and Mrs. W., a married couple from Fort Defiance, Arizona. Mr. W. told me that his grandfather, who was a traditional ceremonial practitioner, tried to teach him his ceremony, but "I never picked up any of his singing ways or any of his teachings. . . . I have no Navajo culture."[19]

When Mrs. W. introduced herself and her husband to me, she was quick to say, "Mr. W. is a Born-Again Christian, but I am traditional."[20] When she excused herself shortly after our interview was underway, Mr. W. mentioned that he was "raised Christian Reform," while "Mrs. W. is a Catholic."[21] When Mrs. W. rejoined the interview, she offered the following by way of explanation for how the family respects their differences in religious preference and health care.

> We've um, we asked for prayer [Christian] requests [when Mr. W. was ill] and because of the way Mr. W. was brought up he chose—I guess it is just an understanding between us, both of us, that he didn't want to practice any type of Navajo religion or have any kind of ceremony performed on him, and uh, so I respected his wishes. . . . I guess it was just kind of like an understanding between the both of us that um we didn't go that route, practice Navajo religion. But to um, try to strengthen our, um to strengthen ourselves with uh with the help of God.[22]

As Mrs. and Mr. W. explain in the following excerpt, their agreement to allow each other to pursue personal choice in this area of life without interference from the other was tested, however, with the onset of parental responsibilities. A critical childhood illness caused them to rethink this arrangement and come to terms with what medical and spiritual options should be sought out in times of need. They told me:

MRS. W.: Like I said, my family is very traditional, we practiced Navajo tradition and we had ceremonies done and um, and Mr. W. respects that. . . . So, I guess the understanding was always that, you know, if the kids got sick, if one of the kids got sick, I always told him that, I would just use every resource that I could to find help if they ever got sick. And I guess, the first encounter that we had was when my daughter, the oldest one was a year old and um she got really sick and she cried like a whole week and couldn't eat, had diarrhea. So, we had [Christian] prayers done on her—.

MR. W.: We took her to a doctor and the doctor couldn't do anything.

MRS. W.: There was really nothing that we could do for her so finally I told him, "I have to resort to the Navajo way, to my tradition." So, we went to go see a crystal gazer [a type of traditional diagnostician]. When we went there he took a piece of glass out of her stomach and then after that she got well and there was nothing wrong—all the sickness that she had, just left her. So, I guess in a way it made him kind of like a believer. But he never really said, "I really believe that," or anything. But, . . . from that day I think he has understood, . . . "If you have to practice the Navajo way, then do it and I won't stand in your way."[23]

This type of situation is not unusual. Other consultants discussed the ongoing commitment it takes to negotiate between divergent belief systems within one family. These decisions are especially complex when children are involved.

Relational Personhood and Malleability

When I saw him I couldn't hug him, I couldn't pick him up because he had all those monitors. They had monitors on him, from his toes to his head. He was just tangled like what you see on the back of your electronic piece of equipment these days. I would just, I just stared at him, and I just totally didn't know what to make of it. And my husband . . . he came up the next day and we both just couldn't believe what happened.[24]

Mrs. J.'s commentary provides insight into the shock and disorientation she experienced after driving into a horse, having an emergency cesarean delivery, and finding herself in an off-reservation hospital with a premature baby tangled in wires. This was certainly not what she had expected to experience with the birth of her first child. With a normal birth in a modern on-reservation hospital, after the Navajo child and placenta are safely delivered, hospital staff bathe the child in warm water, wrap it in a blanket, and hand it to its mother. She shakes her newborn's right hand in greeting, saying, "*Yá'át'ééh shiyázhí*" (Welcome, my son or daughter) to acknowledge to the child and the Holy People that this child is hers.[25] This simple mother–child greeting ritual, part of the love and warmth that Mrs. J. bemoans not being able to share with her newborn son, demonstrates that *Navajo understandings of personhood are relational* rather than autonomous (i.e., they are focused on the collective rather than the individual, as is the case among Euro-Americans).

Underlying this system of belief about relational personhood is the fundamental *principle of synecdoche*; that is, the belief that a detached part of the human body retains lifelong effect. So, the umbilical cord or fingernail clippings can transfer influence to or from the newborn. Thus, toenail clippings or any other such detached parts can stand in for the newborn in a traditional ceremonial or NAC meeting that is conducted while the child is in the NICU and that is aimed at focusing supernatural power on the child's condition and restoring him or her to harmony,.

This principle also means that great care must be taken in disposal of all body parts that detach from the newborn while under the care of hospital staff. Staff members at reservation hospitals and those in the surrounding area who serve Navajo clients must be sensitive to family concerns about the care and disposal of parts of the body important to the safety and future of the child. In the NICU context, concern focuses on the umbilical cord and fingernail or toenail clippings because these are what are used in witchcraft. Members of the child's family must be consulted, however, before any body part is incinerated.

As demonstrated in the mother–newborn greeting, when Navajo people meet for the first time, they divert their gaze downward, extend their right hand, and in a soft voice state their clan affiliations as they very gently shake the other person's hand. *They do not use given or surnames.* Rather, they first say that they are "born of" their mother's clan and "born for" their father's clan. Next, they state the names of their maternal grandfather's clan and their paternal grandfather's clan. A lifelong connection exists between every Navajo and the clans from which she or he descends. By each greeter making these claims, kinship can be established between those first meeting. This means that they will each know what their responsibilities are to each other as dictated by the clan system. Use of kinship terms serves to strengthen the Navajo cultural pattern of relational personhood. And, especially important to the topic of this chapter, the clan system provides enormous support and cooperation to families when in need, including shared parental responsibilities.

In addition, all sisters are co-mothers to each other's children. Thus, when a disabled or other special needs child is born into a family, there are always enough caregivers available because there are a lot of relatives and a lot of "mothers" to help. This also means that if a Navajo mother finds clan relatives among the Navajo staff in an off-reservation NICU facility, she will be very comfortable with them caring for her child—much more so than she will be with non-Navajo personnel doing so.[26]

Whether they are Native American or not, when medical staff give a blood transfusion, perform CPR, or do any other type of treatment to a Navajo infant, they must always take into consideration Navajo notions of relational personhood and the fact that infants are understood to be pliable at birth. Owing to the belief that *Navajo are soft and malleable at birth*, NICU personnel and other hospital staff must take special care when handling Navajo newborns because members of their families who retain this traditional belief will be apprehensive of routine actions altering their neonates' bodies, especially their faces. Moreover, these family members will be especially distraught—as was Mrs. J. —over seeing newborns in NICUs with intravenous lines in their scalps, or any type of device clamped to or pressing on their faces, skulls, torsos, arms, or legs. Her son was hospitalized for an extended period because of his low birth weight and premature status. Understanding her son to be in a malleable state, Mrs. J. was horrified to think that the monitors would permanently influence the shape of her son's face and other body parts. If the newborn subsequently requires surgery, family members will request special assistance in advance to ensure that the procedure is successful.

Protective Prayer before Surgery

> [A] Navajo mother—shocked at seeing her newborn child with cleft lip and palate—may not question the physician's explanation of how the defect occurred, but her lingering question of "why" may not be satisfied until she has reviewed her own prenatal history to account for any breach of tribal prenatal taboos and/or has consulted a Navajo diagnostician.[27]

Most likely, the physician's explanation for the birth defects mentioned in this section's epigraph will be Trisomy 13. In addition to cleft palates or cleft lips, extra digits on the hands or feet are common symptoms of Trisomy 13 worldwide. If a Navajo child were born with other possible defects caused by Trisomy 13, such as close-set eyes (possibly even having the eyes fused together into one), a split or cleft in one iris, or missing skin on its scalp, it would be of grave concern to his or her parents and family. Regardless of the parents' religious affiliation, more than likely some family members would believe the defect was caused by a taboo action on the part of one of the parents during the pregnancy.[28]

Navajo parents of a child diagnosed with Trisomy 13, for example, who lives long enough to be offered facial surgery to repair a cleft lip or palate (most such infants perish quickly), will most likely need to cope with the aforementioned issue of contamination because Navajo surgeons are in short supply. The parents and family will arrange for a prayer to be performed over the child by a traditional or NAC practitioner before the surgery.

The majority of those with whom I spoke who hold traditional beliefs told me of what they termed *protection prayers*. As the name implies, protection prayers are most often done before the medical procedure to protect the patient;

however, as Mrs. M., Dr. A., and Mrs. K.-W. explain below, a second intent is to ensure that the procedure is properly performed.

As Mrs. M. describes, after such a prayer, the *Diyin Dine'é* are compelled to enter the operating room in front of the surgical team, where they will remain throughout the procedure as a divine protective force.

> OK. What usually happens is that if you are going to go through a major surgery, they do a prayer for you, they do a prayer, which is like in my Navajo culture they call it um, *Ach'ą́ą́h sodizin*. Meaning Protection Prayer. OK? . . . A protection prayer is supposed to protect him from anything that will harm. . . . The prayer itself is like to help the doctors, you know. To oversee over the surgery—that the Holy People will all be there before and the doctors will be right behind, you know, and while they do their surgery that everything is to go well. And that's, you know, the kind of protection prayer that they usually do.[29]

Dr. A. clarifies that this protective force is put into place without the knowledge of the biomedical healthcare providers. Their unawareness does not, however, inhibit the efficacy of the Holy People's protective powers.

> It's particularly the case that if someone is going to be undergoing surgery or if it's, if they're going to be undergoing um, uh, like a consultation off the reservation if they are going to go elsewhere for medical care, the patients will often have a ceremony to make sure that everything goes well. And what I was telling you yesterday about the surgeons is that they do not realize the prayers have been said for them too. So that when they come in to do surgery that their hands will be steady and their minds will be clear and they will be able to do a good job. So, it is not just for the patient for his good health, but also for the circumstances of the treatment, you know, and making sure that those people that are applying the treatment are in good shape.[30]

Unknown to the surgeon, the prayer effectively puts into place a protective shield to guide his or her hands. This ensures that no mistakes are made during the procedure. As Mrs. K.-W. describes this:

> The protection prayer, in that case it is called a shielding prayer. See they do the shielding so that there will be a shield, *an invisible shield [is] there to guide the surgeon's hands*. It would be kind of like putting on an extra pair of gloves on you so there is no contact with the person. . . . *That provider actually doing the surgery there would be [encased by] this invisible shield*. So, they will do the shielding prayer for that one ahead of time.[31]

Navajo people following traditional practices are not the only ones providing prayers for infants and other family members destined to undergo surgical procedures. Indeed, Mrs. W. reports how her family uses both Catholic and traditional prayers to protect family members before surgery. She told me:

M. S.: Are there any special preparations that—
MRS. W.: Before?
M. S.: —that you had to have done before you go in for the surgery?
MRS. W.: Yeah. We usually have a protection prayer before and they just pray around that you are going to get well after your surgery or whatever. It is just like the Catholic, they say "Put everything in God's hands, and God will guide the doctor's hand, and then everything will be peaceful within the guidance of God." That is the same way. And then afterwards you can have a Thanksgiving type of a prayer done for you too.
M. S.: Do you know what this type of protection prayer involves?
MRS. W.: It is just a protection prayer. We call it *sodizin, ach'ą́ą́h sodizin*, same thing, protection prayer.[32]

Mrs. H., a self-proclaimed devout Baptist, also told me of a Christian form of prayer used before surgery. While in her case these prayers are firmly rooted in Baptist beliefs, they are based on a similar ideology as that noted by Mrs. W. regarding the Christian notion of surrender to the transcendent God epitomized by the statement: "Put everything in God's hands." As Mrs. H. explains: "We pray for the medical teams, we pray for those working in the health care field—that nothing will go wrong; *that their hands are guided*; and these people were blessed with the knowledge and wisdom to know what to look for, you know."[33] And, increasingly, people call on NAC road practitioners to perform a protection prayer before surgery.[34] After the surgery, when the child has healed, his or her extended family will likely follow up with the Enemy Way when the child is old enough and it is seasonally appropriate to take care of contamination incurred from intimate contact with enemies.

Disability

When the twin boys were about half grown, they were stricken with two diseases which the Night Chant is now used to cure. One was struck blind and the other had both legs drawn up, and, being useless to their mother's people, they were driven out to die. The blind boy took the cripple on his shoulders, to show him where to go, and so throughout the long story they wandered from one cliff-dwelling to

another, begging the hard-hearted *Yei* to cure them. When it became
known that the outcast Dine' were the sons of Talking God, the chief of
all the gods, they were finally cured, but not until the demanded pay-
ment was made.

— Harold Carey Jr., *The Night Chant "The Yeibitchai Dance,"* 2008[35]

A Navajo mother would be culturally prepared to accept a newborn with a physical or mental impairment because disability is a central theme in the plethora
of narratives contained in what are referred to as the Navajo oral histories. It is
especially critical to the story of rejection, redemption, and healing that accom-
panies the Navajo people's most important winter ceremony, the nine-day Night
Way, often called the Night Chant. As pointed out in this section's epigraph, the
oral history of this ceremony features two supernatural heroes known as the
Stricken Twins. They were born to an Earth Surface girl who was seduced by
Talking God.[36] Unlike the Hero Twins (the most famous Navajo supernatural
heroes who were born to Changing Woman), they became malformed: one lost
the use of his legs, and the other lost his vision.[37] The narrative associated with
this ceremony documents how they suffered much adversity along with their
family as they grew up.

To overcome their afflictions, the lame twin climbed onto his blind brother's
back. This allowed him to tell his blind brother where to go, and the two set
out on a quest to find cures for what ailed them. Together, they visited many
Pueblo communities, with no satisfaction. At each location, the *Yei,* or gods,
rejected them; this went on for years. Finally, through perseverance, they
were able to learn all components of the Night Way and to subsequently give
it to the Navajo.[38] This ceremony is known to be exceedingly powerful and
dangerous because it cures the most heinous of all illnesses; in fact, several
who have attempted to learn it have become paralyzed before finishing their
apprenticeships.[39]

Jennie Joe, a Navajo medical anthropologist who has specialized in the study
of disability, notes that the Navajo sociocultural explanations for disabilities
among children fall primarily into two main areas. Congenital abnormalities,
which are present at birth, are usually linked to possible prenatal neglect or abuse
of tribal prenatal rules. Alternately, conditions that occur after birth, during early
childhood, are often seen as evidence of harm directed at the family by someone
inflicting witchcraft on the most vulnerable family member.[40]

Navajo parents and families do not consider disabling conditions such as
blindness, lameness, or slowness in learning how to read to be a form of inadequacy, and the disabled are not discriminated against; rather, they are viewed
similarly to abled children.[41] As Jeanne Connors and Anne Donnellan put it:

Individuals with significant disabilities, whatever their chronological ages, appear to be "frozen in time" between the wide latitude of freedom accorded to youngsters and the assumption of adult duties and responsibilities expected as they end their childhood years and begin the journey to adulthood. It must be emphasized here that individuals with disabilities are not considered "perpetual children" or that no expectations are held for them. Rather, they seem to have reached the critical turning point where they are poised on the brink of assuming adult privileges and duties.... [T]he more able the individual, the more that is expected of him/her; the less able a person is, the more latitude s/he is granted.[42]

Treatment of the disabled is consistent with the Navajo tendency to define individual members of the group according to their unique traits. For example, in the case of developmentally disabled individuals, seizures, running away, or temper tantrums are understood as being a part of that person and are not considered to be either negative or positive qualities, as they would be in Euro-American society. In the Navajo world, such behaviors are simply accepted as presentations of the specific person. This accords with the Navajo concept of health that strives for harmony of mind, body, and spirit and allows even a blind or mentally challenged individual to be considered "cured," regardless of what physical manifestations might still be present.[43] The Navajo Nation is committed to providing the care needed to every child with special needs so that he or she may live in harmony. Toward that end, it has developed a facility offering services for this segment of the community, which is committed to training family members who then can provide care to the child in need, which is the solution preferred by the Navajo Nation.

This is the Growing in Beauty program (GIB), which is specifically designed to meet the needs of Navajo children with delays or disabilities from birth to five years of age while honoring the unique culture and language of the Navajo people. Staff of the program are trained to provide service coordination and direct services, which includes processing referrals from pediatricians, healthcare professionals, and other service providers; providing developmental assessment and evaluation for at-risk children; ensuring that support and services are provided through a team-based approach by early intervention specialists; providing transportation; and offering advocacy and training for families of children in need. Notably, the Navajo clan system works hand-in-glove with the GIB training program. Co-parents and other concerned relatives are trained in order to offer the best possible care to children.

Importantly, GIB personnel also collaborate with staff from off-reservation non-Navajo institutions. These include the Northern Arizona University Institute of Human Development, St. Michaels Association for Special Education, and University of New Mexico Center for Development and Disability.

Predetermined Life Span

> Occasionally, a deformed infant will be abandoned to die, or will be
> brought to a hospital and never taken home again.
> —Alexander and Dorothea Leighton, *The Navaho Door*[44]

As has been stressed throughout this chapter, when faced with a seriously ill newborn or one with major birth defects, Navajo parents, grandparents, and other concerned family members bring their own cultural views and moral tenets into the NICU. In some cases, this can result in serious conflict with medical personnel. A Navajo parent or other relative with traditional leanings watching over an infant in a NICU enduring endless rounds of arduous procedures would likely say, *'iina'al'ąą'téégondiit'ééh*, or "life has different endings." Others might simply say, "let it go." In either case, the individual will mean, "let the disease take its course." In such a case, the parent or other family member is falling back on a lesser known element of Navajo epistemology. It is commonly understood that, "according to one's beliefs, an ideal age exists [for each person]; you are born to live 102 years."[45] I was told that people have traditionally accepted that "there is a time within our life where our time, our number is up, that is where we stop. We don't go beyond that."[46]

Such acceptance is based on the premise that *every Navajo life has a predetermined time span*.[47] Mr. B. explains that this belief applies to newborns as well as adults in the prime of their lives:

> And they say, someone as young as one-day old can only live to one-day old. And that is how it is meant to be. And that is how God intended and that is how God made it that way, and there are some that are lucky enough to reach one hundred years old, old age. That is the intention. So, there is a belief that there is a time, in different stages of your life, everybody has different perimeters that you have to know and accept.[48]

Thus, when faced with the news that their child's condition will not improve in the future, Navajo parents and family members can find peace in the belief that life has different endings and that this is the one predetermined for their newborn. Armed with this ancient knowledge, they can calmly make decisions to withhold or cease treatment for the child.[49]

The medical personnel witnessing this might misinterpret the Navajo parents' action, however. To nurses and other NICU staff, it may appear that the mother or father is not making good medical decisions for her or his child. In such an instance, providers will often involve ancillary support staff such as social workers, the NICU nurses working most closely with the infant, or clinical ethicists. A case conference may be called with the family. Depending on the parents' ages, they may or may not feel comfortable trying to explain their beliefs about a predetermined life span with a group of virtual strangers. In some cases, especially if the Navajo parents have not felt comfortable offering an explanation for their decision, the medical staff will take the more extreme approach of arguing that the child is a victim of medical neglect because her or his family refuses treatment options that they believe will help him or her.[50] Such accusations can result from lack of cross-cultural understanding, as in this hypothetical case of the Navajo infant whose parents refused treatment because it went against a cultural tenet they held dear.

It is not unusual for relatives of the ill child's parents to ask community leaders to come to the hospital to speak on the family's behalf during the case conference. Respected men like Mr. D. do this on a regular basis to explain to biomedical professionals the cultural tenets underlying parental choices. In this instance, the philosophical premise that would most directly influence the parents' decision against aggressive treatment for their newborn would first and foremost be the aforementioned predetermined life span. Notably, as he points out, this tenet simultaneously prohibits the offering of CPR. As he explains:

M. S.: Can you tell me why?
MR. D.: Because . . . if your time is up for the Navajo, then you do the CPR and then the person's heart begins beating again and then later on, and then [that is] kind of like going beyond the point.[51]

In other words, *performing CPR can cause someone to live past his or her intended life plan*, whether the recipient is an adult or a child. This is an important concern. As it happens, however, it is only one of many issues that Navajo people associate with CPR. As will be discussed in the next section, Navajo apprehensions about CPR focus on synecdoche, contamination, and the vulnerability of newborns regarding their developmental stage.

Cardiopulmonary Resuscitation

The infant was not crying like it should. What shall we do? They all were concerned. The Black Wind was asked to perform his ritual on the infant. Black Wind went to the infant and entered into her right foot through her body to the tip of her head. Making a whorl encircled there where he came up. This is where the hair center spot is now, as we see it on our heads. The Blue Wind then went through the hair center spot and came out on the bottom of our toes and our fingers have circle imprints on them. Our muscles also have circle markings on them which we do not know, or see them. This is exactly how it was told long ago. We all can see the imprints on the tip of our fingers and toes. The White Wind went into the infant's left foot and came out where the Black Wind first came out. . . . Yellow Wind entered the infant on the top of her hair center spot and came out on the bottom of her right foot. . . . The infant began to cry faintly.[52]

If a Navajo infant is admitted to the NICU with respiratory problems, which is often the case with premature babies and other sick newborns, and the staff prepares to administer CPR, the child's mother will object if she comes from a traditional family. This is the case for three reasons. First, as will be explained momentarily, the fundamental tenet of Navajo philosophy—synecdoche, the lifelong connection understood to exist between every human and his or her detached body parts—applies to human breath. Second, traditional Navajo view the air most often used for CPR in off-reservation hospitals as contaminated. And, third, Navajo cultural tenets maintain that infants are soft at birth, and that once an infant breathes and cries, the constitution of its body begins to undergo transformation.

According to traditional belief, after the child emerges from the birth canal, internal contact with air through respiration, along with contact between air and the outer surfaces of the child's body, begins to firm the infant. CPR is prohibited in the case of Navajo newborns because the breath most often used in a NICU setting comes from a non-Navajo, which is deemed contaminated because it is that of an enemy. If this breath were to enter the pockets and folds understood by traditional Navajo people to exist inside of every Navajo newborn, it would contribute to a fundamental portion of the child's development and have possible lifelong negative influences on it. This tragic possibility is well illustrated in a sad account shared below by Mrs. S.

Despite Navajo prohibitions against CPR, on occasion in the past, the procedure was administered without the mother's knowledge. The consequences of such a situation are explained by Mrs. S. in the following set of narratives detailing the delivery of a breech birth at a small dispensary in her home community with the assistance of a midwife, a local woman, and two nuns. Mrs. S. believes CPR saved her child's life but caused him lifelong problems. In her own words:

One was mainly a midwife and the other one is just a helper. And these two were just kneeling there on the floor in the delivery room with their rosaries, praying to have that child to cry and here I was just, I can't pray. All I could think is, "I want my child to, oh please." So finally, he cried a small cry, so I don't know back then we never think of CPR that was something that we don't know about. But, that is what she was doing to the baby. . . . But he cried.[53]

The woman who performed the CPR on Mrs. S.'s son was bilaganna. As previously noted, because she is a non-Navajo, or enemy, the bilaganna's breath used in CPR is understood to be a contaminant. Mrs. S. believes that in the case of her son, the procedure—having the breath of a foreigner infiltrate one's body—has had lasting consequences. It deeply penetrated the pockets and folds making up her newborn son's body; as a result, he had severe problems. She explained tearfully, "My son, went into, got into drinking, drugs and out with the wrong crowd. And to this day, he is still in prison in Tucson. And that kills me."[54]

Medical staff coping with a Navajo newborn in respiratory distress will likely believe CPR followed by use of a ventilator to be the best treatment. And this may well be so. NICU staff must be aware, however, that, while *use of ventilator support or of resuscitation done with bagged air (that has not gone through a human body) is not problematic*, as pointed out by Mrs. S., traditional Navajo understandings prohibit the passing of breath from a non-Navajo directly into a Navajo's body.

On the other hand, based on the principle of synecdoche, Navajo individuals avoid *giving* CPR because if the person into whom he or she places his or her breath dies, the recipient's death can have a variety of negative influences on the giver. For example, as pointed out by Mrs. B., in her experience, this procedure causes convulsions.

It happened to my brother. He was a policeman and he shot a man that was running from policemen down at Round Rock [Arizona]. And when that man was dying, they had to use CPR. He [her brother] was breathing in it [the fugitive], and that person died. He was bilaganna. And now, he [her brother] goes into convulsions. And they ah, the crystal gazer and then the hand shaker [Hand Trembler] and then other [diagnosticians] that we know of, you know, how they try to find out what is wrong with him? They said that, "That bilaganna died with your breath, you were blowing in it," and they said, "There is no way we can fix it. You can have an Enemy Way dance for you, still it is in the man that died. Your breath is within him. He died with it."[55]

This fundamental tenet of Navajo philosophy—synecdoche—is also the rationale most often offered by Navajo people for not accepting blood transfusions from non-Navajo people or providing blood for transfusions. As will be discussed next, however, transfusions among Navajo do happen in the modern world, often in NICUs.

Blood Transfusion

> Mrs. J.: Because his blood went down and he was like, but they had to do a transfusion that took like 14 hours because they just can't do it—I guess they can't feed a baby at that weight, you know, just really fast with blood, you have to do it in a slow manner or it takes a lot of time for a preemie to get a blood transfusion. . . . They do it very, very slowly. And it took like 14 hours for him to go through his. . . . There was no time to say no or think about it or let people decide for you. It was just between my husband and I. And decisions had to be made quickly. And so, we did.[56]

As Mrs. J. points out, while she and her husband were alone in a strange hospital without any relatives, her son had to have a blood transfusion in the NICU. Her comment that "There was no time to say no or think about it or let people decide for you" demonstrates that she was unsure about his having this procedure, but she and her husband were in an uncomfortable environment without extended family members and community leaders to whom they usually turn for advice. Mrs. J. is not alone in her apprehension about her son having a blood transfusion. In fact, it is not unusual for Navajo to be apprehensive about this biomedical procedure. In terms of a blood transfusion, medical personnel must ideally work with Navajo family members and use a relative's blood or the blood of another Navajo who has the same blood type as the infant. When I spoke with Dr. A. about this issue, she offered considerable insight.

> I know that transfusions are looked upon askance, a lot of people will refuse transfusions even though their blood count is quite low because you do not know where the blood comes from and if you accept the blood of an enemy then you have *contaminated your own body* and that's very bad. That requires a major ceremony. I know people that have had transfusions and if they're pragmatic about it, if you have to have it, or it has been done, then there is nothing you can do about it later, uh, except to undergo the ceremonies or if those people are not traditional, then um generally speaking they have heard comments about it but then they don't feel particularly one way or the other for themselves.[57]

Dr. A. indicates that concerns over contamination of the body from having the blood of an enemy put into one's body are paramount regarding blood transfusions. This is consistent with what other Navajo people told me. Mrs. Y. simply said, "Accepting blood from another ethnic, you know, group is unacceptable," without elaborating on the matter.[58] Others, such as Mr. T., stressed the difference between the blood running through the veins and arteries of Navajo and that running through the bodies of non-Navajo. Here, blood offered in the form of transfusions is a sign marking the difference between Navajo and non-Navajo, which is of major concern.

M. S.: OK, how about blood transfusions. . . . Are there any prohibitions against having them? I mean taking blood from someone else.

MR. T.: Well, like the same way if you get a blood transplant from another person, it is like from bilaganna and even from Mexican blood, it is a different kind of blood, so it wouldn't work for you. It wouldn't really work for you. . . . That is what they tell us in our traditional, the old people, if you get it from Mexican, then the blood will be different, so it wouldn't work for you. That's what they say.[59]

Echoing this view, Mr. B. Jr. explicates what he understands the consequences of having blood from a non-Navajo in one's system will be to a Navajo: "It will affect you physically and it will affect you mentally. That is just how you are, that is how you are different."[60] Mr. M. Jr. recalled an account told by a friend who said, "My wife, not too long ago when she was having a child, she bled a lot so we have to give her somebody else's blood [from the blood bank] so that she can survive all this and before that she was such a healthy woman. She did everything, but now she says 'I break out in hives. I'm not as healthy as I used to be. I was told not to do these things [meaning have a blood transfusion from the blood bank] when I was a young child. Is this the price that I have to pay? It has an effect on me [that] I don't see as good.' "[61] Without specifying the exact nature of the physical complication that she believed would arise from having such different blood in one's body, Mrs. B. told me: "I never had that one because they have different nationalities, and when they put it in you, and then *you start having problems elsewhere in your body*."[62]

Regarding the mental side of the equation, Mr. D. Jr. noted, "If it is crossing different nationalities, then it gets complicated. . . . It starts haunting you. The person that received the blood transfusion, it's gonna start haunting them. It can't always be cured."[63] It is little wonder, therefore, that blood is only deemed acceptable if it comes from someone "within the same bloodline."[64] This was confirmed by other Navajo with whom I consulted. For example, echoing Dr. A., Mrs. W., a devout Catholic from Pine Springs, Arizona, who practices what she refers to as the traditional Navajo religion, told me that the source of the blood is by far the most critical issue surrounding blood transfusions, rather than the procedure itself.[65] She and her family prefer to exchange blood among themselves when it is needed rather than have family members accept blood from a blood bank.[66]

Like Mrs. W., many Navajo consultants consider blood from relatives to be the best option for transfusions, and other consultants reported having relatives supply blood when transfusions were needed or anticipated.[67] This predilection that transfusion blood come from relatives is nothing new; rather, it has been in place for decades.

> Back in the early '70s when there was a blood transfusion that needed to be done, people used to ask, "Well, can one of my family members donate blood to me instead of just from the blood bank?" They used to be afraid of blood banks because blood bank, you know, you could get blood from they don't know what nationality this person was or what race or whatever. So, they would be more afraid of the blood bank than they were with their family giving their blood to them.[68]

This preference is all fine, well, and good; however, transfusions cannot always be planned. Newborns are often rushed to NICUs, as happened in the case of Mrs. J.'s son, and infants frequently become dangerously ill far from any hospital or clinic. As is described in the following tender story, in such situations, parents may take drastic actions to save their children. This account is shared by a woman who received a transfusion from her father while she was an infant. She told me:

> I am the only one in the family—when I was an infant—that had a blood transfusion. And my dad, until the day he passed away, he wouldn't let me forget, "My blood is what saved your life. I walked with you and I carried you from here all the way to Chinle and caught a ride from Chinle to Fort Defiance [well over fifty miles in distance]." And that is where I was. I guess I had double pneumonia and something else so, you know, I was very thankful to my dad. That he had the courage to walk and that I had the strength to hang on to life until I was given a transfusion. And I got to where I needed to be. So, when he started getting sick, and he started going down, he used to tell me, "I am going down. And my blood is your blood and I don't mean to be boring you with it but that is what kept you going, and I hope you stay strong for me and for many more years to come."[69]

The information presented thus far provides much insight into how Navajo family members draw on cultural beliefs about the body and personhood while

coping with sick newborns in NICUs. In the next section, we turn to the final traditional Navajo tenet that factors in as parents and family members grapple with
a child needing care in such a setting—that is, the generative power attributed to
language. This subject takes us full circle back to the moment in the Navajo oral
histories when the Holy People created their world with song and prayer.

The Power of Language in the Navajo World

> They did a C-section on me at 4:30 AM, but they said, "It is a 50/50
> for both of you because you have lost so much blood and we don't
> know if the baby is going to make it because he is so small and he
> only weighs four pounds, going on four pounds."[70]

In this excerpt, Mrs. J. places special emphasis on how language was a complicating factor in the NICU. In fact, she told me that the most difficult part of
the experience of having her son in the unit was what doctors and other staff
members said to her. As she points out, the words of hospital staff caused her
great concern. She recalls how doctors and nurses—who presumably were following professional standards for care—cautioned her about how factors related
to his prematurity would likely affect her son's physical and mental development.
She noted that such information made her and her husband ill. Her account
sheds light on the debilitating influence such truth-telling can have on Navajo
patients and their loved ones. She reported that she and her family had a traditional ceremony on the second day after the child came home from the hospital.
She said this was done to "give us the faith to look forward believing *we do have a
healthy baby. No matter what the doctors will tell us in the future.*"[71]

To comprehend Mrs. J.'s statement, the *efficacy attributed to language in the
Navajo world must be carefully considered*—based on its role in the oral history, language is understood to have originatory power because it calls things
into being—inclusive of medical conditions. This fundamental belief has direct
applicability to the care and treatment of Navajo patients in biomedical facilities, including neonates. Hospital staff—doctors as well as nurses—working with
Navajo patients must take great care against verbalizing negative prognoses for
all patients, including newborns in NICUs or infants with illnesses having the
likelihood for undesirable complications.

To be explicit and direct in discussions of negative information with their
patients, allopathic providers unintentionally conflict with Navajo values and
ways of thinking, thereby generating tension between themselves and their
patients. Problems can arise with the simple act of gaining informed consent because it requires disclosing the risks of medical treatment or treatment refusal,

which to a Navajo individual can amount to calling these things into being. The complications of truth-telling on the part of biomedical practitioners working with Navajo patients derive from the fact that it requires disclosure of "bad news," or the "truth" of a patient's condition.[72] Mrs. J. was extremely uncomfortable with the language used by medical staff and the fact that her son was inaccessible to her.

Conclusion

The CRC was developed in 1989 to enumerate entitlements and protections intended to be afforded to every child in the world. Although the convention attempted to ensure that the rights of all children would be respected and that all actions dealing with children would be performed in their best interests, this has not always come to pass. The CRC provides well-intended guidelines; however, cultural clashes often occur because the morals and ethics of the families of infants in NICUs and the ethics that medical personnel are trained to uphold differ.

Numerous key beliefs discussed in this chapter factor into the scenario when a Navajo infant is brought into an off-reservation NICU. One of these elements—religious and medical pluralism—encapsulates many of the reasons that it is imperative for healthcare personnel to attend closely to the cultural foundation of Navajo families in the NICU. Regardless of spiritual persuasion, if surgery is called for, family members of the neonate will arrange for protection prayers to be performed by traditional practitioners, NAC roadmen, or Christian clergy. As previously noted, these are done to ensure the success of the procedure as well as to shield the patient from the outsider's negative influence if the surgeon is not Navajo.

Regardless of what denomination any individual may claim, in the Navajo world, healing is a family affair, so traditional beliefs are almost always involved as an underlying frame that must be taken into consideration. All NICU staff should be aware that traditional Navajo concerns over contamination from non-Navajo will dictate decisions on the part of parents of sick newborns to reject CPR or blood transfusions that involve the breath or blood of non-Navajo. Likewise, parents with traditional leanings will prefer that all body parts of the infant that detach while in the NICU be offered to the parents or grandparents rather than incinerated. Family members also may refuse CPR, blood transfusion, surgery, or any other proffered treatment in the NICU because of their core belief in a predetermined life span.

In addition, all NICU staff serving Navajo people should take care to do the following when interacting with concerned parents and relatives of Navajo infants: facilitate the opportunity for every mother to conduct a traditional greeting with her newborn; take great care when handling the newborn because of its perceived malleability; and use caution when speaking to parents and other relatives about the child's condition and prognosis. Navajo people have their own understandings about individuals with developmental delays or disabilities. As discussed earlier, the Navajo Nation's GIB program is specifically designed to meet the needs of Navajo children with these issues while honoring Navajo society. NICU staff should provide the names of any Navajo infants leaving their care who are known to have disabilities or who are at risk for developing developmental delays or disabilities during the first five years of life to the Navajo Nation GIB program.[73]

Notes

1. I am a cultural anthropologist who has conducted research among the Navajo since 1991. I have applied for and received an Ethnographic Fieldwork Permit from the Navajo Nation Historic Preservation Department (NNHPD) before every segment of research conducted on the reservation. NNHPD guidelines require that each "consultant" (the term preferred over "informant," which has connotations of someone sneaking around nefariously) be asked to read (or have read to them) and sign a consultation consent form before an interview begins, that she or he be asked whether or not the information shared could be published by me, what could not be published, and that he or she be given the option to have his or her name used—or a pseudonym selected by the consultant. Most people in my research wanted their names included to give themselves agency for their contributions. It is my understanding that names of consultants are not to be disclosed in this volume; therefore, as in this instance, initials are used for last names, and Mrs. or Mr. is used out of respect. The date is included to anchor the event in time. In the interview excerpts included in the text, M.S. stands for Maureen Schwarz. Wesley Thomas is a Navajo scholar who kindly translated interviews for me.

2. Jing Liu, Xin-Xin Chen, and Xin-Ling Wang, "Ethical Issues in Neonatal Intensive Care Units," *Journal of Maternal-Fetal and Neonatal Medicine* 29, no. 14 (2016): 2322–26.

3. Roy Macleod, *Disease, Medicine, and Empire* (New York: Routledge, 1988).

4. The modern peyote religion, known as the Native American Church (NAC), became formalized in western Oklahoma circa 1880. See Omer C. Stewart, *Peyote Religion: A History* (Norman: University of Oklahoma Press, 1987), xiii. Peyote had been used for millennia in a wide area—from as far south as Oaxaca, throughout central Mexico, and as far north as Santa Fe—as a medicine to be taken internally or applied as a poultice to sores; to foretell future events; to locate lost objects; as a stimulant before warfare or other strenuous activity; and in group religious practices (ibid., 17). While some elements of this religion carried over into the North American version

of the peyote religion, the differences are also significant (ibid., 41–42). The Carrizo originated the North American version of the peyote ritual and taught this religion to the Lipan and the Comanche of the southern plains during the latter half of the nineteenth century (ibid., 49–50). This religion blossomed because of the confluence of peoples and conflicts created by the US government in the establishment of Indian Territory (ibid., 53). From Oklahoma, it spread to the prairies and Rocky Mountain west.

5. Between 2004 and 2007, I conducted research on how Navajo people accommodate biomedical technologies such as amputation, blood transfusions, and organ transplants within the frame of medical and religious pluralism. My findings were published as "I Choose Life": Navajo Perspectives on Medical and Religious Pluralism (Norman: University of Oklahoma Press, 2008). While conducting this project, I sought information on any beliefs about health, healing, or the body that Navajo people currently held that derived from a Christian faith or the NAC rather than traditional precepts. I discerned none that would pertain to infants in NICUs.

6. Ethelou Yazzie, Navajo History, volume 1. Navajo Curriculum Center (Rough Rock, AZ: Rough Rock Demonstration School, 1971), 9.

7. Ibid., 17.

8. Aileen O'Bryan, The Diné: Origin Myths of the Navaho Indians. Bureau of American Ethnology, Bulletin 163 (Washington, DC: Government Printing Office, 1956), 112.

9. Interview with Mr. D., July 11, 2004.

10. Edward Said, Orientalism (New York: Pantheon Books, 1978), 54.

11. Interview with Dr. A., June 10, 2005.

12. If contamination results from contact with the death of a Navajo or surgery that is performed by a Navajo physician, the Evil Way can be performed to rectify the situation (interview with Mr. D., June 22, 2005).

13. John Adair, Kurt Deuschle, and Clifford Barnett, The People's Health (Boulder: University of Colorado Press, 1988), 22; Stephen Kunitz, Disease Change and the Role of Medicine (Berkeley: University of California Press, 1983), 131; Gladys Reichard, Navaho Religion: A Study of Symbolism (New York: Pantheon, 1950), 84.

14. Dorothea Leighton and Clyde Kluckhohn, Children of the People: The Navaho Individual and His Development (Cambridge, MA: Harvard University Press, 1947), 15.

15. Alan Waxman, "Navajo Childbirth in Transition," Medical Anthropology 12 (1990): 192–93.

16. Rita Begay, Navajo Childbirth. Ph.D. dissertation, Department of Public Health, University of California Berkeley (Ann Arbor, MI: University Microfilms, 1985), 91; Alan Waxman, "Navajo Childbirth in Transition," Medical Anthropology no. 12 (1990): 194–98.

17. The cited statistic on the profound shift to hospital births is from W. T Boyce et al., "Social and Cultural Factors in Pregnancy Complications among Navajo Women," American Journal of Epidemiology 124 (1986): 242–53. Despite this trend, traditional techniques for assisting births and caring for newborns and mothers have not been forgotten. Indeed, many such practices are presently incorporated into the birthing

experience in modern hospitals across the reservation. Ibid., 187–203; interview with Mrs. K.-W., August 10, 1992; George Hardeen, "Hogans in Hospitals: Navajo Patients Want the Best of Both Worlds," *Tribal College* 5, no 3 (1994): 20–24; Maureen Hartle-Schutte, "Contemporary Usage of the Blessingway Ceremony for Navajo Births," Master's thesis. American Indian Studies (Tucson: University of Arizona, 1988).

18. Native Americans—including the Navajo—remain colonized peoples today. Thus, the assumption of medical control over Native American bodies was and is an expression of the power relationship of what some refer to as "internal colonialism." Patricia Kaufert and John O'Neil, "Analysis of a Dialogue on Risks in Childbirth," in *Knowledge, Power, and Practice*, ed. Shirley Lindenbaum and Margaret Locke (Berkeley: University of California Press, 1993), 50. Given changing and emerging federal Indian policies, scholars and politicians suggest use of the term *neocolonialism*. The term *post-colonialism* does not apply to the current American situation, however, because the 2.4 million Native Americans currently living within the boundaries of the United States remain a conquered people.

19. Interview with Mr. W., June 21, 2005.

20. Interview with Mrs. W., June 21, 2005.

21. Interview with Mr. W., June 21, 2005.

22. Interview with Mrs. W., June 21, 2005.

23. Interview with Mr. and Mrs. W, June 21, 2005.

24. Interview with Mrs. J., July 3, 2005.

25. This information comes from the following sources: Ursula Wilson, "Traditional Child-Bearing Practices among Indians," in *Life Cycle of the American Indian Family*, ed. Janice Kekahbah and Rosemary Woods (Norman, OK: American Indian and Alaska Native Nurses Association Publishing Company, 1980), 20; Rita Begay, *Navajo Childbirth*. Ph. D. dissertation, Department of Public Health, University of California Berkeley (Ann Arbor, MI: University Microfilms, 1985), 117; and an interview with Mrs. A., July 29, 1991. Similarly, at a home birth, following safe delivery of the placenta, the child was bathed in warm water, wrapped in a blanket or sheep pelt, and handed to his or her mother, who would greet the child while shaking his or her right hand. Irene Stewart, *A Voice in Her Tribe: A Navajo Woman's Own Story* (Socorro, NM: Ballena Press Anthropological Papers, no. 17, 1980), 11; Ursula Wilson, "Traditional Child-Bearing Practices among Indians," in *Life Cycle of the American Indian Family*, ed. Janice Kekahbah and Rosemary Woods (Norman, OK: American Indian and Alaska Native Nurses Association Publishing Company, 1980), 20.

26. Jennie Joe, "Cultural Influences on Navajo Mothers with Disabled Children," *American Indian Quarterly* 6, no. 1/2 (1982): 170–92.

27. Ibid., 170.

28. Birth defects such as a newborn being born with extra digits on the hands or the feet were traditionally understood as being caused by the making of a weaving fork while pregnant (interview with Mrs. K., August 4, 1992). See also Flora Bailey, "Some Sex Beliefs and Practices in a Navajo Community: With Comparative Material from Other Navaho Areas. Reports of the Ramah Project," *Papers of the Peabody of*

American Archaeology and Ethnology 40, no. 2 (Cambridge, MA: Peabody Museum, 1950), 41. This follows the Navajo adage that the nature of an illness or problem contracted by a child while in the womb is patterned after the cause; that is, like produces like. In the 1940s, Bailey was told that if a pregnant woman cut or sawed the edge of an old cooking pot, for example, the child would be born with a cleft lip (ibid., 41, 42).

29. Interview with Dr. A., June 11, 2005.

30. Interview with Dr. A., June 10, 2005.

31. Interview with Mrs. K.-W., July 5, 2005.

32. Interview with Mrs. W., June 17, 2005.

33. Interview with Mrs. H., July 14, 2005.

34. This was reported in independent interviews with Mrs. M. on June 11, 2005 and Mr. L. on July 13, 2005.

35. The full reference is Harold Carey Jr., "The Night Chant 'The Yeibitchai Dance.'" *Navajo People, Culture, and History* (February 15, 2008), accessed October 14, 2017, http://navajopeople.org/blog/the-night-chant-the-yeibitchai-dance/.

36. Gladys Reichard, *Navaho Religion: A Study of Symbolism* (New York: Pantheon, 1950), 93, 128, 137.

37. Navajo attitudes toward twins have fascinated outsiders for some years. Claims have been made over the years that Navajo do not like having twins, that one usually dies during the first year of life, and that one twin will be abandoned to die. Jerrold Levy's work on the subject found these all to be unsubstantiated rumors. He found post-neonatal mortality rates to be significantly higher among twins than among single births, and some evidence of a circumstantial nature that tends to substantiate the belief that parents of twins tend to neglect one member of the pair. Jerrold Levy, "The Fate of Navajo Twins," *American Anthropologist* 66, no. 4 (1964): 883–87.

38. Gladys Reichard, *Navaho Religion: A Study of Symbolism* (New York: Pantheon, 1950), 51, 54, 58, 68, 485.

39. Ibid., 82, 94–95.

40. Jennie Joe, "Cultural Influences on Navajo Mothers with Disabled Children," *American Indian Quarterly* 6, no. 1/2 (1982): 186.

41. The concept of a child in Navajo culture is one of approaching, being, and becoming. Before the age of 6 or 7, a Navajo child can virtually do no wrong and is allowed great freedom in exploring his or her world in an experiential way. This permissiveness reaches an abrupt end at age 6, when parents begin to insist on appropriate behavior and to teach the child the duties and responsibilities of an adult. Jeanne Connors and Anne Donnellan, "Citizenship and Culture: The Role of Disabled People in Navajo Society," *Disability and Society* 8, no 3 (1993): 270–71.

42. Ibid., 271.

43. Ibid., 270.

44. Alexander Leighton and Dorothea Leighton, *The Navaho Door* (Cambridge, MA: Harvard University Press, 1945), 61.

45. This was told to me on several occasions, for example, in interviews with Mr. D. on August 11, 1993; Mr. D. on June 11, 2004; and Mr. D. on June 22, 2005.

46. Ibid.

47. Interviews with Mrs. J. on July 3, 2005 and Mrs. S. on June 6, 2005.

48. Interview with Mr. B. on June 16, 2005.

49. Alexander Leighton and Dorothea Leighton, *The Navaho Door* (Cambridge, MA: Harvard University Press, 1945), 61.

50. Thomas Cunningham, "A Life Below the Threshold?" *Narrative Inquiries in Bioethics* 6, no. 1 (2016): 63.

51. Interview with Mr. D., June 22, 2005.

52. Excerpt from an unpublished transcription of an interview with Mr. Curley Mustache, an esteemed Navajo elder by Jones van Winkle. Tsaile, Arizona. Manuscript in author's possession, 1970.

53. Interview with Mrs. S., June 15, 2005.

54. Ibid.

55. Interview with Mrs. B., July 15, 2004.

56. Interview with Mrs. J., July 5, 2005.

57. Interview with Dr. A., June 10, 2005.

58. Interview with Mrs. Y., June 14, 2005.

59. Interview with Mr. T., June 28, 2005.

60. Interview with Mr. B. Jr., June 16, 2005.

61. Interview with Mr. M. Jr., June 13, 2005.

62. Interview with Mrs. B., June 10, 2005.

63. Interview with Mr. D. Jr., June 15, 2005.

64. Ibid.

65. Interview with Mrs. W., June 17, 2005.

66. Ibid.

67. Interview with Mrs. Y., June 14, 2005.

68. Interview with Mrs. K.-W., July 5, 2005.

69. Interview with Mrs. M., June 11, 2005.

70. Interview with Mrs. J., July 3, 2005.

71. Ibid.

72. Joseph Carrese and Lorna Rhoades, "Western Bioethics on the Navajo Reservation Benefit or Harm?" *Journal of the American Medical Association* 274, no 10 (1995): 826.

73. The Growing in Beauty program can be reached at P.O. Box 1420, Window Rock, AZ 86515 or 928-871-6338, or 1-866-341-9918, and more information is available at http://www.nnosers.org/growing-in-beauty.aspx or http://www.nnosers.org/gib-az-nm-brochure-1-.pdf (accessed on September 22, 2018).

10

Moral Status and Care
of Impaired Newborns

An African American Protestant Perspective

Patrick T. Smith

One of the most challenging situations in neonatal health care that many have faced, whether families or healthcare professionals, is how one perceives and cares for severely impaired newborns with a very limited life expectancy. This issue became much more stark in my own mind through two different experiences. The first was serving in an unofficial role of "counselor" to an Asian American pastor and his wife who had just received the news that their unborn son was diagnosed with a fatal heart disease. The prognosis was that their son would only live an agonizing day or two without multiple very extensive, invasive, and expensive surgeries. And if they opted for these multiple very extensive, invasive, and expensive surgeries, maybe their son would only live a few months. They were getting pressure from family members as well as some people in health care that they should not continue with the pregnancy because there is no value in a life like that. And so the choices presented to them were at the extremes. Either you do all you can for this child after he is born, which would be expensive, painful, and more than likely produce suffering (with the implied connotation that you don't want to do that, do you?) or you go ahead and terminate the pregnancy now.

This particular couple was very unsettled about these options and this way of framing the issue. They were not comfortable with the idea of abortion and wanted to affirm the value of their son as a gift from God, but they also did not want to prolong any suffering that he may experience while dying. They heard that I had done some work in end-of-life ethics and that I oversaw the ethics department for a hospice. After a few weeks of contemplative prayer with their church community and waiting on results from other medical tests, I connected them with some skilled pediatric hospice professionals. These skilled caregivers were able to develop a plan that allowed this family and their church community to affirm the full and high moral status of their son while not unnecessarily prolonging the dying process. Their son lived several months without all the surgeries. He also had some meaningful interactions with his older brother and extended family during his brief life. The family was able to make some precious memories. For me, this case illustrated how important it is that parents and medical professionals understand that a child can be highly valued at the same time as not doing everything medicine can do in order to sustain the child's life.

This theme re-emerged in a second experience that occurred while I was serving on a hospital ethics committee. This time, the family was African American. We were discussing a case, again about a severely impaired newborn with a limited life expectancy. Many folks on the care team wanted the family to stop treatment because they thought that by continuing, they were causing harm. Other professionals disagreed. There were a few additional mitigating factors in this case, the details of which are not as important as the statement of one doctor as she was walking out of the room. She said, "We're always going to have these kinds of problems in neonatal care if we don't dislodge the thinking that all lives are equally valuable in these situations. They are not."

I did not have the opportunity to interact further with her because she left the meeting for another appointment. Many other professionals in the room did not agree with her assessment. However, I was deeply unsettled by this comment. Upon reflection, I was aware that the historical context of African Americans' encounters with health care and the many challenges facing African American neonates and their mothers' reproductive health played a significant role in my discomfort. I certainly understood her aversion to the tragic consequences of these situations. But I didn't and still do not think the problem is where she placed it. I also understood that the form of African American Christian tradition I embrace would want to affirm the high and full moral status of these precious little ones with a limited life expectancy while at the same time not unnecessarily prolonging the dying process or causing more harm just for the sake of preserving life.

This chapter addresses the question of moral status and care of severely impaired African American newborns from the perspective of African American Protestant Christian theology and spirituality. The vantage point from which I engage with this topic is what is known as the black Christian tradition. In speaking in this seemingly unified way, I do not want to give the impression that the black Christian tradition is singular or monolithic. It should go without saying that it is very diverse. It comprises many denominations, including a myriad of Baptists, Methodists, and Pentecostals such as the Church of God in Christ, just to name a few. Also, there are various theologies represented, and each of these theologies often has various sociopolitical philosophies and spiritualities. Nevertheless, there are some minimal features that are widely recognized by those who self-consciously identify with this expression of Christian faith as it emerged:

> Out of the crucible of racial oppression . . . as a nonracist appropriation of the Christian faith. As such it represented the capacity of the human spirit to transcend the conditions of racism in both thought and practice. In addition, this tradition has been represented as a fundamental principle of criticism justifying and motivating all endeavors by blacks for survival and social transformation. Thus the black Christian tradition has exercised both priestly and prophetic functions: the former aiding and abetting [black people in their] capacity to endure the effects of racism, the latter utilizing all available means to effect religious and moral reform in the society at large.[1]

The black Christian tradition, so understood, strives to live out both the spiritual and social implications of its faith by drawing creatively and imaginatively from the rich resources of the larger Christian tradition for the purposes of community empowerment and uplift. I count myself as part of such a tradition. A central unifying claim of this tradition is its anthropological principle, which tenaciously insists on the equality of all people "under God regardless of race or any other natural quality" or social location.[2]

In keeping with the prophetic dimension of the tradition, in the first part of the chapter, I describe the impact of racism and class as co-determinants of disparities concerning health outcomes among African American women and their newborns. Aspects of the priestly dimension appear in the second half of the chapter. There, I seek to identify how theological and spiritual resources deeply embedded within this tradition should inform our thinking on the moral status of seriously impaired African American newborns and the medical decision-making implications that follow.

Insights from the Prophetic Aspect of the Black Church Tradition

Healthcare Disparities and African American Neonates

There have been significant advances in medical care for newborns, such as "newer antibiotics for infections, respirators and pharmaceutical treatments for immature lungs, and advanced electronic monitoring" and a decreasing infant mortality rate since the 1950s.[3] Despite all of this, there remain deep disparities between blacks and whites in the area of neonatal care. These inequities are well established and widely known. For my purposes, it is helpful simply to highlight one grouping of inequities related to neonatal care: the racial dynamics regarding rates of infant mortality among black and white infants in the United States, premature births, and the associated health challenges for African American newborns with respect to low birth weight.

To begin, the United States has the distinction of being one of the countries with the lowest infant survival rate among industrialized nations. Further, "the decline in infant mortality has not been the same for all racial groups."[4] In particular, "African-American infants have a 2.4-fold greater mortality rate than non-Latino white infants."[5] African-American normal-birth-weight babies (those weighing at least 2,500 grams) still "are substantially more likely to die before their first birthday."[6]

Related to this is another alarming aspect of this discussion. It is the data surrounding *low birth weight* (LBW) and *very low birth weight* (VLBW) of black infants. "LBW is a leading determinant of first-year mortality risk and the primary factor underlying the racial disparities in [infant mortality rates]."[7] The occurrences of LBW (babies weighing between 1,500 and 2,500 grams) and VLBW (babies weighing less than 1,500 grams) for infants are associated with a higher mortality rate. Before going further, it is important to note that in the LBW and VLBW groups, the infant mortality rates and the chances of survival for these infants, whether black or white, are relatively the same.

Strikingly, though, there is a substantially larger percentage of black infants born in these groups than white infants. "Black infants are born in the LBW group at a rate that is almost 2 times that of white infants. Black infants in the VLBW group are born at this weight at a rate that is 2.6 times that of white infants."[8] Even those LBW black infants who do survive are at increased risk for facing many enduring health challenges. According to Collins and David, LBW "is closely linked to serious long-term physical, mental, and emotional disabilities." In referring to the extant writings on the issue, they go on to say: "An expanding body of published literature shows that LBW is also a major risk factor for several chronic diseases of adulthood, including coronary artery disease and type II diabetes."[9] The potential lifelong health challenges resulting from LBW are immense.

Genetic Explanations of Healthcare Disparities?

Yet, many remain unclear as to the underlying mechanisms that can explain such stark discrepancies. In order to explain such glaring differences in black and white birth outcomes, some suggest the problem is genetic. The idea behind this explanation is to see the category of race as based in human biology. In other words, according to this view (also known as biological realism), the concept of race depicts real, objective categories in the biological nature of distinct communities of human beings. Appeal is made then to these fixed biological traits found in different "races" to explain the prevalent racial healthcare disparities.

Apart from the deeply troubling ethical issues with such a view, this approach to explaining the disparities in birth outcomes is mostly rejected on empirical bases. Summarily speaking, with respect to genetic science, "the genes that create [the] differences in surface appearance are so few compared to the genes that create the structural and functional similarity among all humans that they have little association with important biologic characteristics."[10] This is true regardless of those areas where there is a higher correlation with particular health challenges and specific ethnic communities. For example, concerning the occurrence of hypertension and diabetes among African Americans being two to three times higher than among whites, Kawachi and co-authors write:

> But it is a gross oversimplification to assume that differences in genetic susceptibility could explain the observed racial disparities. For instance, representative surveys of populations in West Africa and African-origin populations in the Caribbean have revealed prevalence rates of hypertension and diabetes that are two to five times lower than those of black Americans or black Britons. Such observations alone should give pause to molecular enthusiasts who have advocated for the vast expansion of research efforts to search for the genetic explanation of racial disparities in these diseases.[11]

Empirical work on this topic indicates that "human genetic diversity appears to be a continuum, with no clear breaks delineating racial groups." Further, and more central to the aims of this chapter, there is no clear sense of the "role that specific genes play in several of the birth outcomes that contribute significantly to racial and ethnic disparities, such as LBW or prematurity."[12]

Socioeconomic Status Explanation of Healthcare Disparities

Others have suggested that socioeconomic status best explains the disparities in birth outcomes. The problem lies in risk factors related to social disadvantages and lower socioeconomic status for many African American women during pregnancy. The issue, then, is *not* primarily about race. A number of studies do explore this very important hypothesis. Analyses along these lines regarding the poor birth outcomes of African American women tend to "focus on differential exposures to protective and risk factors *during pregnancy*, such as current socioeconomic status, maternal risky behaviors, prenatal care, psychosocial stress, or perinatal infections."[13] The idea is that if you could include the proper protections and otherwise correct for the risk factors, this would erode some of the disparity that exists between black and white infants.

However, the results, according to studies by Collins, Wu, and David, are that "maternal factors and conditions during pregnancy—age, education, marital status, income, parity, interpregnancy interval, cigarette smoking, and impoverishment—failed to account for the African-American infants' birth weight disadvantage."[14] Coming to a similar conclusion, Lu and Halfon find that the disparities in birth outcomes cannot be accounted for sufficiently based on the kinds of risk factors mentioned above for women *during* pregnancy.[15] So, it would seem that socioeconomic status cannot do *all* the explanatory work.

The general direction of the evidence suggests that both racism and socioeconomic status often work together in mutually reinforcing ways to perpetuate disparities in health.[16] Nazroo and Williams suggest that social and economic inequalities, as well as the effects of racism, can be viewed as fundamental causes of ethnic inequities in health.[17] Thus, they must be understood in tandem as potential co-determinants. Nevertheless, we must be careful not to collapse the issue of race into the category of socioeconomic status or "class" as if the latter does all the work in explaining the disparities with which we are dealing. Race and socioeconomic status remain distinct categories with distinct issues and distinct outcomes even if they are connected to each other in important ways. Donald A. Barr surveys a number of studies that look at the effect of race on health outcomes after accounting for socioeconomic status. The conclusion these studies draw is that blacks still had more unhealthy outcomes than their white counterparts.[18]

Systemic Racism and the Life Course Perspective as an Explanation of Healthcare Disparities

Let us consider another alternative in order to explain the negative birth outcomes with respect to African American women's offspring. Interestingly, increasing numbers of health professionals are taking seriously the hypothesis that conditions of chronic stress experienced by many pregnant African American women over their life course, as a result of systemic racism, are a significant contributing factor to neonatal health inequities and to African American women's health status. The ongoing works of Richard J. David, James W. Collins, Michael C. Lu, and Neal Halfon, among others, have been particularly insightful on this score. Over the years, they have researched this public health problem in depth. They hypothesize in one way or another that "chronic maternal stress, accumulated across the life course and across generations, could explain the increased risk of preterm birth observed in disadvantaged social groups."[19]

Some of these researchers have proposed that understanding "the high rates of African American infant mortality in the United States requires analysis of the effects of race as a social construct. . . ."[20] In order to better appreciate this hypothesis, we need to understand what is meant by this concept. To say that "race" is a social construct is to highlight that it is an idea developed around a social imagination and set of practices that appear to be natural but are actually the creation of a given society. *Race*, then, is an invented social category that divides human beings into hierarchical groups based on differences in physical appearance, geographical origin, and ethnic backgrounds.[21] Historically speaking, as Alyssa Ney points out, "the system of racial classification is designed to enforce a social hierarchy, with [those who are considered] white people at the top."[22] This is just what it meant to be white in addition to one's ethnic heritage—be it Polish, Germanic, Scottish, and so forth. To be *racialized*, then, is "to be systematically subordinated or privileged, in virtue of being perceived as 'appropriately occupying certain kinds of social position.' "[23]

For some, of course, such a Life Course hypothesis is controversial. Nevertheless, these factors do have explanatory power with respect to explaining the stark disparities on birth outcomes. Moreover, there are many aspects of this view that deeply resonate with the lived experiences of those who might identify with African American Christianity or the black church tradition. It is the kind of empirical data presented here that informs the social ethics of this particular faith community in relation to neonatal and women's health care. To bring some of this together, I briefly expand on two key aspects of the hypothesis.

First, it takes into consideration the basic trajectory and accumulation of experience across the life spectrum. In other words, it highlights that "pregnancy is not an isolated event independent of prior life experiences."[24] Michael Lu and Neal Halfon describe such an approach to include the *impact on* and *experiences of* African American women being racialized. They write:

> Racism can take multiple forms; it can be internalized, personally mediated, or institutionalized. It can manifest itself as discriminatory medical care. Several studies have documented that African Americans receive less ambulatory, hospital, and disease specific care than do Whites and experience greater barriers in their interactions with the medical care system. It can also manifest itself in residential segregation. Greater Black–White gap in infant mortality has been found in cities that are more segregated. Exposure to racial discrimination is not limited to pregnancy, but extends across the lifespan. The effect of race on birth outcome is likely mediated in part through this weathering of racism and racial discrimination over the life course.[25]

This life-course approach takes into account the effects of chronic stress on the reproductive process. Part of the complex biochemistry of pregnancy under usual circumstances is the production of stress hormones. Moreover, there are many stressors that often are associated with pregnancy (e.g., concern about delivering a healthy baby, nervousness about the process of delivery, anxiety about becoming a first-time parent). Some researchers have gone beyond these stressors *during pregnancy* to see what role chronic social stressors might play in explaining racial disparities in birth outcomes. They examine and analyze the effects of chronic stress produced by racism and other socially disadvantaged considerations on a pregnant woman's body system and organs.

Lu and Halfon "hypothesize that the higher rate of preterm delivery among African American women is related to not only stress exposures during pregnancy, but more important stress response that has been patterned by lifelong exposures to chronic and repeated stress."[26] These researchers are seeking to identify the relevance of additional stress hormones that are produced by those "chronic social stressors that are pervasive in the everyday lives of many African American women." This would include things like discrimination on the job, economics, housing, lack of resources in one's community, and safety, among numerous others that might be identified.[27] Of course, these kinds of social stressors are not relegated only to communities of ethnic and racial minorities. Many others find themselves in similar situations where they, too, would experience many of these same chronic social stressors.

Yet, we need to remember that the approach taken here sees both race and socioeconomic status as co-determinants, not as co-extensive, of some of the health disparities we are considering. The point, then, the authors seem to be making is that living in a racialized society may further exacerbate for racial minorities, in some cases, the common problems experienced by other women who share the same socioeconomic status or, say, disadvantaged conditions. They argue that these kinds of ongoing conditions over an African American woman's life course and the corresponding wear and tear on the body that is produced thereby increase the allostatic load to a level that can negatively affect birth and other health outcomes by triggering the delivery process prematurely. This, according to Lu and Halfon, is a significant contributing cause of "racial disparities in birth and other health outcomes."[28]

A second relevant observation to highlight is that these effects are intergenerational. This means that the "factors, experiences, and exposures experienced by one generation . . . relate to the health of the next generation."[29] In relation to the disparities in birth outcomes, Collins, Wu, and David expound this point in the following way:

We previously found that the birth weight patterns of African-American infants with African-born mothers and White infants with US-born mothers are more closely related to one another than to the birth weights of African-American infants with US-born mothers. Consistent with this finding, studies have shown that African-American infants of Caribbean-born mothers also weigh more than African-American infants of US-born mothers independent of maternal risk status during pregnancy. These observations suggest that inter-generational factors closely related to lifelong minority status contribute to the African-American women's reproductive disadvantage.[30]

If these data are sound, then the consequences of all of this should arrest our moral attention. All of this suggests that there is something about growing up as a black female in the United States that has a detrimental impact on her repro-ductive health. This serves as a partial explanation for why some well-educated and high-socioeconomic-status African American women still experience a disparity in premature births, LBW babies, and infant mortality compared with their white counterparts. This further evidence suggests that the issue of negative birth outcomes of African American women is not best explained by consider-ations of socioeconomic status or expressions of personal responsibility *only*, on one hand, or by genetics, on the other. (If it were genetic, we would expect similar birth rates of offspring from mothers of color born in Africa and the Caribbean to that of US-born African American mothers' offspring, which we do not see.) It seems it would be important for neonatal caregivers to be aware of how racism and African American women having lifelong minority status in the United States might be affecting their childbearing health and their offspring.

Bearing Witness—Behind the Data Stand Real People

We must be careful to remember that behind the troubling statistics and seem-ingly ever-expanding data stand the material lives of real people. John Hoberman reminds us that "the recitation of endless statistics documenting medical racial disparities depersonalizes the human dimension of what is happening to black people." He goes on rightly to identify that the consequences of the "sheer mag-nitude of the African American health disaster can produce both emotional de-tachment and a dehumanizing sociological reduction of black life to its bleakest essentials." [31] Hoberman here is echoing the insightful analysis generated over sixty years ago by the social critic James Baldwin in his book *Notes of a Native Son*. There is a memorable passage contained therein concerning black hu-manity, where Baldwin writes:

[They are] a social and not a personal or human problem; to think of [them] is to think of statistics, slums, rapes, injustices, remote violence; it is to be confronted with an endless cataloguing of losses, gains, skirmishes; it is to feel virtuous, outraged, helpless, as though his continuing status among us were somehow analogous to disease—cancer, perhaps, or tuberculosis—which must be checked, even though it cannot be cured.[32]

The systemic dimension of racism naturally leads to the dehumanization and depersonalization of people of color in terms of how they are *viewed* within a racialized imagination and *treated* in a racialized society. And yes, the list of the statistics and data about the inequities African American women's health and reproduction outcomes introduced is longer, much more comprehensive, and more nuanced than described here. The thrust of this part of the chapter is not to recite or rehearse these in any great detail, despite appearances to the contrary. Instead, I raise these issues to underscore that the disparities in this area of neonatal care constitute a major public health problem and are a major concern that African American Christianity and spirituality seek to address—not only in the context of neonatal care but also outside of it.

The prophetic aspect of the black Christian tradition identifies *and evaluates* the larger social conditions as violating the way God wants human communities to be and interact with each other in order to flourish. This concrete social reality is to reflect a kind of covenant relationship that is to be characterized by righteousness and justice. This is emphasized while never losing sight of the lived experiences of people. In this sense, biblical texts that inform this social vision call the community of faith to "embody the uniqueness of the covenant relationship to God in concrete social arrangements."[33] This vision takes its cues from the biblical prophets who spoke truth to power structures, both political and religious, which perpetuated injustices.

> He has showed you, O mortal, what is good; and what does the LORD require of you but to do justice, and to love kindness, and to walk humbly with your God?
> —Micah 6:8

> Give justice to the weak and the fatherless; maintain the right of the afflicted and the destitute. Rescue the weak and the needy; deliver them from the hand of the wicked.
> —Psalm 82:3–4

> But let justice roll down like waters, and righteousness like an ever flowing stream.
>
> —Amos 5:24

Informed by empirical data, it is a primary role of the prophetic aspect of the African American Christian tradition to display prominently those unjust conditions and social arrangements in order to prick and motivate the collective conscience of society toward alternative visions of doing life together. It is the community's responsibility to bear witness to this social vision. Resources from this tradition have been a source of inspiration *and hope* for African American Christians to be resolute in their attempts to reveal the fundamental dehumanizing depths of racism and its connections to the negative psychosomatic health effects of racial segregation and discrimination.[34] More positively, the tradition bears witness in that it affirms that all of humanity is made equally in the image of God. Dr. Martin Luther King Jr. repeatedly appealed to this theological idea in order to firm up one's sense of "Somebodyness." The idea of humanity being made in the image of God served as a divinely inspired counterpoint "in the wake of questionable sociological and biological analyses of the 'Negro' plight."[35]

Insights for Professional Neonatal Care from the Prophetic Dimension

It is appropriate for neonatal healthcare professionals to ask, "What difference does all this make with respect to our work in a neonatal intensive care unit (NICU)?" It would seem that some of these insights are outside the purview of the particular context of a NICU. While many neonatal healthcare professionals may be troubled by the data, how might all of this make an impact on the care they provide in their professional spaces? Reflecting on the insights from the prophetic dimension of African American Christianity described here, I want to suggest that these insights might *broadly* inform the work of neonatal healthcare professionals in the following way. The prophetic dimension of African American Christianity contributes to expanding neonatal healthcare professionals' moral imaginations by reminding them that attention must be paid to the unethical and dehumanizing "causes of the causes," so to speak. This aspect of African American Christianity is a reminder that injustices in human relationships are not merely relegated to the interpersonal level only but are also reflected in social, systemic, and institutional relations. This contribution allows clinicians to have "eyes to see and ears to hear" these realities when they may have been previously unaware. It reminds all of us that we must look beyond interpersonal dynamics to begin to address these kinds of disparities. Further, clinicians can develop more creative possibilities in addressing these problems within their sphere of influence.

Approaching race as a social construct pushes us beyond what some call the "commonsense" understanding. It moves us to think about these issues much more systemically. The "commonsense" way of thinking about the issue can be described in the following way. "Person A (usually, but not always, white) consciously, deliberately, and intentionally does something negative to Person B (usually, but not always, black or Latino) because of the color of his or her skin."[36] Alternatively, to see racism as systemic injustice, we need to understand it as a cultural phenomenon. That is:

> [A] way of interpreting human color differences that pervades the collective convictions, conventions, and practices of American life. Racism functions as an ethos, as the animating spirit of U.S. society, which lives on despite observable changes and assumes various incarnations in different historical circumstances. Analyses that focus only or principally upon interpersonal dynamics (what person A does to person B) miss the more important and pivotal cultural setting that not only facilitates such acts, but makes them understandable and intelligible.[37]

A recent essay by a group of healthcare professionals echoes these points. These authors implore health professionals to take a more active role in addressing the larger systemic issues that are the root causes of premature deaths "for different races despite the best efforts of individual health care professionals."[38] They argue that, given their relative power and privilege as clinicians and researchers, there exists an ethical responsibility to dismantle structural racism, considering its direct impact on health. They highlight that the health problems produced by structural racism "are causing widespread suffering, not only for black people and other communities of color but for our society as a whole." Structural racism in health care "is a threat to the physical, emotional, and social well-being of every person in a society that allocates privilege on the basis of race."[39] Here, they are echoing the words of Dr. Martin Luther King Jr.'s idea of a Beloved Community.

For those willing to pick up the mantle with respect to this issue, they offer four recommendations. First, healthcare professionals need to make a concerted effort to learn about, understand, and acknowledge the history of racism in the United States. Second, clinicians should pay attention to how racialized imaginations have shaped narratives about disparities and informed their implicit biases. Third, as noted previously, it is essential that there be a deeper understanding of race and racism in its full social dimensions. And last, they encourage research and clinical practices that "center at the margins" in order to achieve equity.[40] This means a shift in viewpoint that does not normalize the white experience that is "informed by centuries of explicit and implicit racial bias."[41] This last point is significant and perhaps the most difficult aspect of their recommendations, given the moral vision and political will necessary to achieve it. One can get a sense of the depth and breadth of this recommendation, when they write:

Centering at the margins in health care and research will require re-anchoring our academic and health care delivery systems—specifically, diversifying the workforce, developing community-driven programs and research, and helping to ensure that oppressed and under resourced people and communities gain positions of power. Centering at the margins in clinical care and research necessitates redefining "normal." We can do so by using critical self-consciousness—the ability to understand how society and history have influenced and determined the opportunities that define our lives. For clinicians, that means reflecting on how they arrived at their understanding of a diagnosis or clinical encounter and being willing to understand how patients arrived at theirs. Centering at the margins not only provides an important opportunity to practice more patient-centered care but can also generate new findings and clinical insights about the experiences of people who are often overlooked or harmed by our institutions.[42]

In some ways, this chapter is an attempt to implement some of these distinct recommendations. I am very aware that this requires a paradigm shift of sorts in the minds and practices of neonatal care professionals. To be sure, this is only a meager beginning. If all of this is right-headed, then the point is clear. If we want to care for this vulnerable population of severely impaired African American newborns, then we must care about eradicating structural racism.

Insights from the Priestly Aspect of the Black Church Tradition

In light of these troubling realities, how might the black Christian tradition inform our understanding of the moral and religious status of premature infants and severely impaired newborns with a very limited life expectancy? This part of the chapter appeals to theological and spiritual resources that (1) inform an understanding of the moral status of severely impaired African American newborns, (2) provide a framework for an approach to dying and death helpful for NICU settings, (3) explain why a commitment to the sanctity of life does not entail medical vitalism, and (4) highlight some Christian practices and other resources for those in NICUs.

Moral Status and the Image of God

The anthropological principle of the black Christian tradition would want to affirm the *high* and *full* moral status of severely impaired newborns with a limited life span. Not only do the conceptual resources seem to move in this direction, but also the sociohistorical background of African American neonatal care and the Christian tradition's emphasis on love provide the motivation to do so. This claim is based on the theological understanding of the image of God and the ethical implications that flow from it. In Christian tradition, this is what grounds the *high* and *full* moral status of people, what affirms their value and worth regardless of who they are, where they are from, what they believe (or don't), or what they do. It is difficult to understate the significant role that the theological notion of the *image of God* has played in an ethical approach to life that is informed by Christianity. It is a powerful idea that historically has fostered movements of liberation. It has proved significant for supplying the theoretical underpinnings that drive emancipatory change in the world by encouraging people influenced by resources from within this tradition to value, respect, and protect all human beings.[43] The consequences of these resources can be seen in movements that address issues of poverty, liberating people experiencing the ravages of different sorts of oppression and mistreatment, advocating for human and civil rights for people of various backgrounds in various circumstances, and so forth.

Of course, there are different ways this idea has been unpacked in various Judaic and Christian traditions. In keeping with the purposes of this volume and my authorial assignment, I here offer a particular *Christian* framing of the idea that I suggest deeply resonates with many African American expressions of Christianity. It is one that stresses the embodied nature of humanity. It is an approach that emphasizes the role of Jesus in understanding what the image of God means and its implications for both living and dying. On this way of framing the topic, the point of reference for understanding the *image of God* is centered in the public life and teachings of Jesus of Nazareth. So, for African American expressions of Christianity, Jesus becomes a centralized figure and symbol of the ethical life. This is critical to appreciate.

To understand better what many Christians sometimes mean by the phrase *image of God*, it is important to get a sense of how Christian texts seem to present this idea and some theological reflections that have resulted from it. When an object is said to be an "image" in biblical writings, it means a special *connection* to something in a manner that may also involve *reflecting* it. For example, in the biblical book of Daniel 3, both of these notions, connection *and* reflection, are at work in the story of King Nebuchadnezzar building a large image of himself. In that context, images were constructed to represent earthly kings, and they could also stand for a representation of various gods. These images were constructed "in order, to establish their presence as rulers where they were not physically present." They were *connected* to the king in such a way that disrespecting them meant disrespecting the king himself. Moreover, these images are in some way intended to reflect that which they represent. These images also were supposed to mimic attributes similar to the original. So in the case of King Nebuchadnezzar in Daniel 3, the great height of the image is meant to represent his power and the gold his vast opulence.[44] Hence, the ideas of special connection and reflection are central to a proper understanding of what it is for one thing to be an image of something else, theologically speaking. It is this "connection *and* reflection" association that provides insight into what it means for Christian tradition to understand humanity as being in the *image of God*.

To unpack this further, we need to note how the *image* language in Christian scriptures is applied to Jesus in a distinct way from its application to all other humans. The New Testament identifies Jesus as being *the* image of God. Without going into sustained and in-depth exegetical analyses due to space limitations, here I simply highlight two Christian texts to establish the point. The first is 2 Corinthians 4:4. It describes Jesus as being *the* image of God. This verse, situated in a context that discusses spiritual blindness, makes the claim that the glory of God is remarkably and distinctly displayed in the glory of Jesus. The language of the two (God and Jesus) as being related in this way describes connection, while the emphasis on the glory that is shown through Jesus as proper to God shows that Jesus *reflects* what he is *connected* to—namely, God.[45]

Another significant text is Colossians 1:15, which portrays Jesus of Nazareth in just as lofty a manner. It describes Jesus as "*the image* of the invisible God." The exalted theological context in which this verse rests highlights the church's poetic confession of faith concerning the primacy of Jesus. The description of God being invisible in Christian tradition raises a crucial theological issue concerning the knowledge of God. How is it that God can be known when God is inaccessible to the senses? The answer is found in this highly developed theological understanding of Jesus. In short, the claim from a widely accepted interpretation of Jesus in Christian tradition, though not universal, is that Jesus is so *connected* to and *reflects* the invisible God that He gives people the opportunity to see God. This widely accepted confession of Christian faith proves significant. The important consequence for the claims being made in this section is that Jesus, the totality of his life, is identified as *the* image of God.

This understanding of the image of God takes the body and embodied experiences seriously. The value and worth of humans is not found in some abstractions rooted in, say, mental capacities, expressions of moral agency, sentience, and so on. The biblical text of Genesis 1:26–28 states that all other people, men and women and everyone along the spectrum regardless of age or ability, are made *according to* the image of God. People bear a special relation of reflection and connection to Jesus and, hence, God. "Because people in their entirety, including their bodies, are in God's image, particular bodily characteristics never warrant ascribing greater worth to one race, ethnicity, or gender over another."[46]

The devaluation of groups based on these criteria is complex and morally problematic. The black Christian tradition calls on society to work for more just social realities. However, people deserve more than the application of some abstract notion of justice. Given their special connection to and reflection of God, people deserve love. From this angle, it becomes evident that love then entails expressions of justice in concrete, material ways. It is love that "generates true solidarity, fellowship, interdependence, inclusive community, and unified mission." This radical, inclusive vision of God's intended relationships between people based in love means that:

> [P]eople with special needs due to disabilities warrant special care and welcome. They have an image-based dignity that does not waver, regardless of their ability or potential ability. [Jesus], God's image, models God's embrace of disability on the cross and through a resurrected but wounded body. All of humanity shares in such woundedness and vulnerability in a variety of forms—physical, mental, moral, spiritual—without losing the dignity of being... in the image of God. Whoever would treat those with disabilities as God does must view them in terms of their destiny as well as their dignity—in terms of God's intention for them to be a divine reflection as well as their special connection with God.[47]

These resources deeply inform the understanding of and motivation behind the affirmation of the *full* and *high* moral status of severely impaired African American newborns with a limited life expectancy in light of the sociohistorical context of African American neonatal care.

The Sanctity of Life Principle and a Theology of Dying and Death

The image of God in humans is the key Christian doctrine that is said to underpin the ethical core of the sanctity of life principle. The sanctity or inviolability of human life historically has emerged as a key moral principle in conversations concerning end-of-life medical ethics. Given the nature of this project, however, I focus primarily on how the Christian resources identified previously inform a particular understanding of the sanctity view. Moreover, I submit that the appeal to the sanctity of life with respect to care for severely impaired African American newborns ought not to entail vitalism and that there are theological reasons for rejecting it.

Traditional formulations of the sanctity or inviolability of human life prohibit "intentional killing of human beings for reasons incompatible with justice."[48]

Many advocates of the view further highlight the implications of the sanctity principle *for* end-of-life medical ethics. They affirm on one end of the spectrum that "it imposes . . . an absolute *negative* obligation, namely an obligation to *refrain*" from such killing that is incompatible with justice. And on the other end of the spectrum, the sanctity of human life "imposes no unqualified positive obligation to seek to prolong life in all circumstances."[49] Three broad theological themes help provide a framework for understanding and applying this middle-ground implication of the sanctity of life view and its relevance for end-of-life neonatal care.

The first theme is that Christian tradition has affirmed that death is a foe or an enemy to be resisted, to be sure. But, theologically speaking, death is a defeated enemy. Throughout the tradition's writings, death is a foe in that it is associated with negative emotions like fear, despair, and anguish. "The snares of death encompassed me; the pangs of Sheol laid hold on me; I suffered distress and anguish" (Psalm 116:3). Numerous other texts from Christian tradition depict death as a natural process that comes after a faithful life journey regardless of how that life ends. Psalm 116:15 reads, "Precious in the sight of the Lord is the death of his faithful ones." Death is also depicted in the biblical texts as the entryway for a future reward for faithful service. And so death is sometimes seen as something that should not always be resisted.

Herein is the theological tension that death is depicted, in some ways, as both friend and foe.[50] According to Christian theology, death is not final. First Corinthians 15:21 reads, "For as by a man came death, by a man has come also the resurrection of the dead." The idea of the resurrection, however understood, is often considered the great hope of the Christian faith. Therefore, when thinking about severely impaired newborns, Christian tradition carves out a middle path between two extremes. "Because the medical profession is trained to heal and thwart death, there are clearly times when heroic measures have gone way beyond the point of benefit and have unnecessarily prolonged life or even caused greater suffering. Refusing to allow death to come in the course of time is every bit as much 'playing God' as attempting to control the timing and means of death" through various forms of euthanasia.[51] The idea here is that to embrace *this* earthly life as the highest good or as something that has absolute value to be hung onto at all costs can easily slide into a form of idolatry.

Second, "suffering is a challenge to persevere in and an opportunity to overcome."[52] On one hand, the Bible speaks of suffering as producing something of value in the lives of people. Just as Jesus endured physical pain on the cross that brought him closer to the "mystery of his sacrifice," physical suffering, for example during an illness, can draw people closer to God. This idea has been formulated in different ways in Christian tradition. While suffering can be framed in a manner that has profound meaning, we must tread very carefully when it comes to suffering and the role of Christian religion. It is not clear that severely impaired newborns are able to frame their experiences in such meaningful ways. Nevertheless, like others with severe cognitive disabilities, infants in grim situations are still known by God.[53] Further, the faith community can draw near to God in such situations when they embody spiritual practices of accompaniment, presence, and compassionate palliative care to journey with these precious, even if severely disabled, little ones.[54]

Nor should the idea be taken to mean that people should not work to alleviate the actual suffering of others and the conditions that cause suffering. Christians "have a mandate to remove or reduce suffering, despite the fact that patients [or their loved ones] can find meaning in it."[55] This obligation is central to the Christian faith. Jesus is often held up as an example on this point (Mark 1:32–34). While many Christians believe in the healing power of God, they do not always expect to be healed from their illnesses. It would be presumptuous to think otherwise. Regardless, there are limits to the types of interventions that can be employed to eliminate or reduce suffering. "Suffering is a part of human life and there will always be disease and deterioration that presents challenges to Christians as to others."[56] There are sicknesses unto death. Faith traditions are helpful in these stages of life because they offer social connection and structures by which people find meaning in suffering. African American spirituality sees Jesus as standing with those whose backs are against the wall.[57] This theological point helps us to identify the balance between two extremes. The first extreme is to think of suffering as an unqualified evil that must be eradicated at all costs, even if that means employing euthanasia in cases of Trisomy 13 or 18, Tay-Sachs disease, or Lesch-Nyhan syndrome. The other extreme is a too-rigid acceptance of suffering that leads to unnecessarily prolonging death and the experience of suffering.[58]

The third theme is that Christians live in the tension of divine providence and human stewardship. In Christian tradition, God is thought to be continually at work in the affairs of this world. The black Christian tradition has affirmed this idea in that God is seen as one who ultimately fulfills God's purposes compatible with loving justice and expressing compassion in the world. Those in this tradition can thereby have and maintain hope as they simultaneously work for a better tomorrow. It is this way of thinking about providence and human responsibility that underlies the often-quoted, and sometimes misapplied, statement by Dr. Martin Luther King Jr. that, "even though the moral arc of the universe is long, it bends towards justice."[59] The context of the quote does not support a kind of blind historical determinism. The theological driving force behind this public statement for Dr. King is based in God's loving and just character, vision for humanity as seen in Jesus, and providential work through people exercising moral agency. In a real sense, those in this faith community affirm that God is in control. Yet, within the black Christian tradition, this is never understood in isolation from people acting in the world. In an equally real sense, the faith community affirms that they make real decisions that have real effects in the world.

Medical technology and its proper use is just one such area where people must make choices while ultimately leaving the results up to God. These are often tough choices that in fact affect the timing of death. Robert Orr and Susan Salladay vividly describe this point when they write:

> Dying is a process. Sometimes this process happens quickly. . . . But more often in today's era of intensive medical care, dying happens slowly. When we consider the use of ventilator support to help a person breathe, dialysis to replace failed kidneys, transfusion to replace blood loss, antibiotics to replace infections, CPR to try to reverse cardiac arrest, we see that the timing of death can involve an element of choice. Whether a patient dies in a few minutes, or a few hours, or a few days, or a few weeks is often determined by a choice about whether to start, continue, or stop one or more of these treatments.[60]

These choices are unavoidable. God's providence and human action work together. "Humans are called to be caretakers and decision-makers who must exercise wisdom in the use and allocation of all the resources that God places into [their] hands."[61] Most advocates of a properly nuanced and theologically informed sanctity view are aware that in a medical context, there are situations in the process of dying where it is morally appropriate to either discontinue current treatment or refuse it altogether. Though mathematical precision cannot be had with respect to determining exactly when this is the case, many proponents of the sanctity view embrace a couple of widely accepted notions that can provide some assistance. And they generally take these to be right-headed.

First, "physicians have no obligation to provide [nor patients to receive] pointless and futile or contraindicated treatment."[62] Second, and more important for this context, life-sustaining medical treatment can be withheld or discontinued and should not be considered obligatory if there is no realistic hope of recovery, if treatment becomes excessively burdensome, or if the burdens outweigh the benefits.[63] This includes a family's decision about their severely impaired newborn. In such situations, one can refuse "treatment that would prolong . . . life for [an indefinite] period of time if that treatment really does carry with it significant burdens."[64]

Sanctity of Life Does Not Entail Medical Vitalism

This way of framing the sanctity principle theologically stresses a middle ground between two extremes. And many, though not all, of those who embrace the sanctity or inviolability of human life would deem various forms of euthanasia in cases of Trisomy 13 or 18, Tay-Sachs disease, or Lesch-Nyhan syndrome as being incompatible with the principle. They would also, on a Christian understanding of the view, reject forms of unnecessarily prolonging the dying process of severely impaired newborns. Christian tradition affirms a deep-seated respect for this life. But we must be careful not to worship it. Such is said to be the basic thrust of the sanctity view.

It is important that the sanctity view be distinguished from and explicitly contrasted with two other schools of thought sometimes at work in conversations surrounding end-of-life medical ethics. They are the Quality of Life view and the Medical Vitalist view. Some expressions of the Quality of Life view make a value judgment about the worthwhileness of the patient's life. This view holds that certain lives drop below a particular threshold because of disease, injury, or disability that devalues these patients' lives. In other words, certain lives are not worth living. If so, then the level of moral obligations could be diminished toward these people. Some conclude on this basis that it is not wrong to end these lives intentionally, whether by act or by deliberate omission, in order to bring about death. [65]

It should be clear that this view does not accord well with an approach that seeks to affirm the full and high moral status of severely impaired newborns. One implication of the image of God doctrine is that people are valuable in virtue of their humanity. Their lives are not any less valuable simply because they may have some sort of disease, injury, or disability. The black Christian tradition would affirm that severely impaired newborns still have full moral status even if it is very clear that they have an extremely limited life span. So, it would not be consistent with the sanctity of life view to *speak* of severely impaired newborns as having lives that are no longer or not of any value or are of minimal value, as some versions of the Quality of Life view might suggest.

This is important for neonatal healthcare professionals to appreciate, even if they do not agree with the value judgment regarding these patients. If nothing else for those who do not share the view, it should nevertheless encourage caution as to how quality of life considerations are *stated* with respect to severely impaired newborns in general, and given the context of African American newborns in particular. African American parents, family members, clergy, and others who are in community with severely impaired newborns cannot be faulted for being highly suspicious of, and perhaps even resistant to, quality of life language used in reference to their loved one. This is especially the case if we take seriously the dehumanizing role that racialized imaginations and racism play in producing and often maintaining conditions across the life spectrum of African American women's lives that contribute to such negative birth outcomes, as suggested by a number of researchers. The claim being made here is *not* that there is no place for a *particular kind* of quality of life judgment. This is discussed in more detail later. However, it is to suggest that if the judgment is made with respect to the value of the patient, then this will be in tension with the view being developed here.

On the other end of the spectrum is the Medical Vitalist view. It holds that this human life is of *absolute* moral value—the sort that requires it to be preserved at all costs. The reasoning behind this school of thought is:

> Because of its absolute worth, it is wrong either to shorten the life of a patient or to fail to strive to lengthen it. Whether the life be that of a seriously disabled new born baby or an elderly woman with advanced dementia, vitalism prohibits its shortening and requires its preservation. Regardless of the pain, suffering or expense that life prolonging treatment entails, it must be administered.[66]

Unfortunately, the Medical Vitalist view is often confused with the notion of the sanctity or inviolability of human life. Or, it is sometimes thought that the sanctity or inviolability view entails a vitalist understanding of human life as described previously. I want to claim that these are distinct and in some ways incompatible views, theologically speaking, and should be understood separately. One critic of the sanctity or inviolability of life view straightforwardly writes, "From the equal value of human life follows 'vitalism,' or the view that all lives must be prolonged equally regardless of whether such [life-sustaining treatment] measures will benefit or harm a particular patient." The reason for the claim that medical vitalism flows from the sanctity or inviolability view is that one ends up using "the language of benefits or burdens to a patient" in order to help make the decision to discontinue life-sustaining treatment. According to such critics, this assumes—"explicitly or implicitly—a quality of life approach."[67] Hence, those who embrace the sanctity principle are being inconsistent in its application because, presumably, they "affirm the equality of all human lives and yet base arguments for a limited duty of life-preservation on implicit quality-of-life considerations."[68] These judgments are thought to be incompatible, though my claim is that this is not necessarily the case.

Certainly, the sanctity view holds that all human lives are equally valuable. This is not controversial. Also, I think we need to acknowledge that there is language adopted by proponents of the sanctity view that employs benefits-and-burdens criteria and the patients' interests when thinking about refusing various forms of life-sustaining treatment, as stated earlier. This is where it becomes crucial to identify what is meant by the phrase "quality of life" in the context of end-of-life neonatal care.

Following John Keown, there are two ways that quality of life language can be understood and employed. Only one of them, in the end, is inconsistent with the sanctity of life view. Highlighting an important distinction between the worthwhileness of treatments and the worthwhileness of the patient can assist in appreciating the difference between the two senses. According to Keown:

> A treatment may not be worth while either because it offers no reasonable hope of benefit or because, even though it does, the expected benefit would be outweighed by burdens which the treatment would impose. . . . Notice, however, that the question is always whether the *treatment* would be worth while, not whether the patient's *life* would be worth while. Were one to engage in judgments of the latter sort, and to conclude that certain lives were "not worth living," one would forfeit any principled basis for objection to intentional killing.[69]

It is within these parameters that it is appropriate to employ, I think, *qualified* quality of life language. This could be considered the distinction between, say, "Quality of Life" (capitalized) considerations that refer to a school of thought concerning the value of human life, and "quality of life" (lowercase) considerations that focus on the benefits or burdens of a given treatment. Another way of putting this is that "quality of life" is "used to refer to an assessment of the patient's condition as a preliminary to gauging the worthwhileness of a proposed treatment."[70] Often in a medical context, many who hold to the sanctity of life view do make appeal to quality of life considerations in this second sense. In such cases, though, the quality of life considerations are aimed at the treatment in relation to the potential health outcomes of the patients and not at the value of the patients themselves. Again to quote John Keown, "For, in order to decide whether a proposed treatment would be worthwhile, one must first ascertain the patient's present condition and consider whether and to what extent it would be improved by the proposed treatment. The exercise is often described as involving an assessment of the patient's quality of life now and as it would be after the treatment."[71]

The distinction is often confused in medical and ethical discourse. When this happens, it can potentially cause problems in terms of communication and assessing the reasons for moral justification behind certain decisions at the end of life. Some would rather do away with quality of life language altogether and just speak about benefits and burdens to the patient. We must also acknowledge, however, that the language is firmly entrenched, such that we need to be clear about its the possible range of meanings in order to minimize misunderstandings. The point here is simply that quality of life considerations understood with respect to the worthwhileness of the treatments pose no threat whatsoever to maintaining the equal value of all people regardless of medical condition, as espoused by the sanctity principle.

206 RELIGION AND ETHICS IN THE NICU

Having said all of this, it must be kept in mind that human life, theologically speaking, is a *basic* good, not an ultimate or an absolute one. Those who rely on these sorts of theological resources and those critics of the sanctity view must not confuse the notions of what it is that makes human life *valuable* and what it means to *flourish as human beings*. To be sure, these are integrally related, yet they are not the same. While innocent human life should never be ended intentionally, according to the sanctity view, there is no moral obligation on Christians to continue *merely* to sustain biological life at the end of life when it is clear in view of our best available judgment that severely impaired newborns with a very limited life expectancy (who remain inherently valuable nonetheless) will not ever be able to exemplify other human values that contribute to human flourishing, theologically understood.[72] I want to suggest that by distinguishing the basis of human value from human flourishing and correctly understanding how *qualified* quality of life considerations are applied in a medical context, those who espouse a sanctity view in the NICU can consistently reject medical vitalism while maintaining a robust principle of the sanctity of human life.

Christian Practices and Other Resources for Dying Well Enough: Opportunities and Obstacles

Of course, these theological parameters are certainly tested when confronted with the devastating realities of various diseases and genetic disorders such as Trisomy 13 or 18, Tay-Sachs disease, or Lesch-Nyhan syndrome and the suffering they inflict on the family unit. This is where these families may indeed find some support as the Christian community engages in particular practices that embody their values. However, it must be acknowledged that sometimes faith communities do not adequately embody their values in ways that are meaningful and helpful to their members who have suffered the loss of an infant in the NICU. This is where neonatal healthcare professionals can play a very important role. Based on quantitative and qualitative studies, a significant number of Christian families "perceived that their greatest sense of community was derived from hospital staff."[73] Regardless, there is a central place for Christian communities to practice their faith in the NICU.

Other contributions from the Protestant tradition in this volume have suggested and detailed a number of Christian practices that accompany the dying. My alignment with African American Protestantism can certainly incorporate many of these other Protestant traditions' spiritual activities in the NICU. Nevertheless, I want to emphasize the interdependence of three important practices that are central to African American Christian experience—namely, prayer, song, and the reading of the Bible—which are likely to be practiced by African American Christians in the NICU.

The significant role of prayer cannot be overemphasized. There may very well be calls for God to bring healing at the bedside. As alarming as this may be to some NICU professionals, given babies with such conditions as Trisomy 13 or 18, Tay-Sachs disease, or Lesch-Nyhan syndrome, this should not be always, and perhaps in most cases, understood as an obstacle to making important decisions for whatever time the family has with their severely impaired infant. In many cases, the prayer for healing is thought of as an affirmation of faith that these issues are in the hands of God. It is an affirmation that when medicine and professional health care have let people down, God does not. In this tradition, "healing is achieved through prayer." Even if there is not a cure or a miraculous turnaround of events, healing can still take place. It is thought that prayer is healing.[74]

One way this healing happens is through the important role of lament as a form of prayer and song. Lament gives way to hope—as informed by biblical narratives—in the face of suffering and hardship. When the Psalms are prayed, they expose the deep-seated and raw emotions families experience in the face of their suffering and mourning of their infants' condition, instead of hiding them. In this process, people are able to "bring before God the raw intensity of the emotions evoked by death."[75] Related to this is a close relationship between song and prayer. "Both are deep expressions of the [African American's] understanding of God in light of the problems of evil and suffering."[76] The Psalms or songs of lament furthermore serve as a reminder of the value of God's gift of life. It is not uncommon to hear worship songs or well-known hymns of the church being sung just before entering into prayer. These songs can have a comforting effect as people turn to God in prayer in light of the hardships they experience in coming to grips with the condition or death of their infant. The process of lament through song also serves as a springboard for the need of divine mercy.

The hospice philosophy of care as developed by Dame Cicely Saunders needs to be an increasing resource for African American Christians in compassionately caring for their severely impaired newborns. Many African Americans underutilize hospice in general. Neonatal professionals need to appreciate why there may be resistance to neonatal hospice care for severely impaired African American babies. For some in this community, there is a sense that they have been systematically excluded from the benefits of American health care. So, when neonatal care professionals strongly emphasize palliative care measures only as opposed to other more aggressive therapeutic options, it could come across as another form of marginalization. This is not to say that it should not be offered or that professionals should shy away from these conversations. The important issue is that neonatal care professionals should speak carefully and be patient given the sordid history described in the first half of this chapter. It is just as important for clergy, other faith leaders, and members of faith communities to understand the benefits of pediatric hospice care and the theological compatibility of pediatric hospice care with their faith, and to be able to communicate each of these to the communities they serve.

Conclusion

By way of conclusion, it was one of the goals of this chapter to foster a better appreciation of the challenges some racial minority communities face when engaging professional health care. Further and more specifically, religion has historically played a vital role not only in helping African American communities to cope but also in empowering them to resist the dehumanizing challenges produced by various forms of racism when it has emerged in our society. To be sure, the African American intellectual tradition is multifaceted and includes various forms of nonreligious humanism. Religious resources are only one part of this rich tradition. Yet, they remain a very important part and continue to play a vital role in the communities who embrace them.

Nothing that has been communicated in this chapter would suggest that there is an unconditional deference to the religious views of the patient–family dyad in all end-of-life neonatal healthcare situations.[77] I want to claim that there are better and worse ways of reasoning from the conceptual resources within religious traditions, as is the case with any other nonreligious theoretical approaches that inform communal practices. I argue that neonatal healthcare professionals should seek to understand how these resources might be at work and why. The patient–family dyad whose medical decisions are informed and influenced by religion should not be cavalierly dismissed. Taking these resources seriously acknowledges the complex landscape in which people make medical decisions.

Considerations Neonatal Caregivers Should Keep in Mind

- Be aware of the sordid legacy of racism in the United States, which often informs why some communities mistrust healthcare systems when in professional spaces.
- Pay attention to how racialized imaginations have shaped narratives about healthcare disparities.
- Be intentional about "centering at the margins" in order to achieve greater forms of equity in health care.
- Recognize that, although the black church tradition's anthropological principle supports a version of the sanctity of human life that would affirm the

full and high moral status of severely impaired newborns, this does not mean that life is to be preserved at all costs, no matter the amount of suffering experienced. Preservation of this earthly life is important but not the highest good. Medical vitalism is to be rejected on this basis.

- Be careful as to how one articulates quality of life considerations with respect to the care of severely impaired African American newborns.

Notes

1. Peter Paris, *The Social Teachings of the Black Churches* (Philadelphia: Fortress, 1985), 11.
2. Ibid.
3. Donald A. Barr, *Health Disparities in the United States: Social Class, Race, Ethnicity, and Health, Second Edition* (Baltimore: Johns Hopkins University Press, 2014), 127.
4. Ibid.
5. James W. Collins Jr. and Richard J. David, "Racial Disparity in Low Birth Weight and Infant Mortality," *Clinics in Perinatology* 36 (2009): 63.
6. Barr, 129.
7. Collins Jr. and David, 64.
8. Barr, 129.
9. Collins Jr. and David, 64.
10. Barr, 96.
11. Ichiro Kawachi, Norman Daniels, and Dean E. Robinson, "Health Disparities by Race and Class: Why Both Matter," *Health Affairs* 24, no. 2 (March/April 2005): 343–44.
12. Michael C. Lu and Neal Halfon, "Racial and Ethnic Disparities in Birth Outcomes: A Life-Course Perspective," *Maternal and Child Health Journal* 7, no. 1 (March 2003): 23.
13. Ibid., 13.
14. James Collins Jr., Shou-Yien Wu, and Richard J. David, "Differing Intergenerational Birth Weights among the Descendants of US-born and Foreign-born Whites and African Americans in Illinois," *American Journal of Epidemiology* 155, no. 3 (2002): 210.
15. Lu and Halfon, 13.
16. Kawachi, Daniels, and Robinson, 343–52.
17. James Y. Nazroo and David R. Williams, "The Social Determination of Ethnic/Racial Inequalities in Health," in *Social Determinants of Health*, 2nd edition, ed. Michael Marmot and Richard G. Wilkinson (New York: Oxford University Press, 2006), 238–66.
18. Barr, 120–27.
19. Richard J. David and James W. Collins, "Layers of Inequality: Power, Policy, and Health," *American Journal of Public Health* 104, no. S1 (2014): S9.
20. Ibid.

21. Barr, 91.
22. Alyssa Ney, *Metaphysics: An Introduction* (New York: Routledge, 2014): 265.
23. Ibid.
24. Collins, Wu, and David, 210.
25. Lu and Halfon, 23.
26. Ibid., 22.
27. Ibid., 22.
28. Ibid., 22.
29. Collins Jr., Wu, and David, 210.
30. Ibid.
31. John Hoberman, *Black and Blue: The Origins and Consequences of Medical Racism* (Berkeley: University of California Press, 2012), 5.
32. James Baldwin, *Notes of a Native Son* (Boston: The Beacon Press, 1955), 25.
33. Bruce C. Birch, *Let Justice Roll Down: The Old Testament, Ethics, and Christian Life* (Louisville, KY: Westminster John Knox, 1991), 176.
34. See Emile M. Townes, *Breaking the Fine Rain of Death: African-American Health Issues and a Womanist Ethic of Care* (New York: Continuum, 1998).
35. Richard Wayne Willis, Sr., *Martin Luther King Jr. and the Image of God* (New York: Oxford University Press, 2009), 116.
36. Bryan N. Massingale, *Racial Justice and the Catholic Church* (New York: Orbis, 2010), 13.
37. Ibid., 15.
38. Rachel R. Hardeman, Eduardo M. Medina, and Katy B. Kozhimannil, "Structural Racism and Supporting Black Lives—The Role of Health Professionals," *New England Journal of Medicine* 375 (December 1, 2016): 2113–15, accessed May 15, 2018, doi: 10.1056/NEJMp1609535.
39. Ibid., 2113.
40. Ibid., 2113–15.
41. Ibid., 2114.
42. Ibid., 2114.
43. John F. Kilner, *Dignity and Destiny: Humanity in the Image of God* (Grand Rapids, MI: Eerdmans, 2015), 6.
44. John F. Kilner, "Special Connection and Intended Reflection, Creation in God's Image and Human Significance," in *Why People Matter: A Christian Engagement with Rival Views of Human Significance*, ed. John F. Kilner (Grand Rapids, MI: Baker, 2017), 141–42.
45. Ibid., 143.
46. Ibid., 157.
47. Ibid., 156–57.
48. Luke Gormally, "Terminal Sedation and Sanctity-of-Life in Medicine," *Terminal Sedation: Euthanasia in Disguise?* ed. Torbjorn Tannsjo (Dordrecht, The Netherlands: Kluwer, 2004), 87.
49. Ibid.

50. Dennis P. Hollinger, "A Theology of Death," in *Suicide: A Christian Response*, ed. Timothy J. Demy and Gary P. Stewart (Grand Rapids, MI: Kregel, 1998), 258–61.

51. Ibid., 260.

52. Ibid., 261.

53. John Swinton, *Dementia: Living in the Memories of God* (Grand Rapids, MI: Eerdmans, 2012).

54. For an excellent essay on practicing compassion with dying children within a faith community, see Tonya D. Armstrong, "Practicing Compassion for Dying Children," in *Living Well and Dying Faithfully: Christian Practices for End-of-Life Care*, ed. John Swinton and Richard Payne (Grand Rapids, MI: Eerdmans, 2009), 139–62.

55. Karen Lebacqz, "Redemptive Suffering Redeemed: A Protestant View of Suffering," in *Suffering and Bioethics*, ed. Ronald M. Green and Nathan J. Palpant (New York: Oxford University Press, 2014), 269.

56. Ibid.

57. Howard Thurman, *Jesus and the Disinherited* (Boston: Beacon, 1976).

58. Hollinger, 263–64.

59. Martin Luther King Jr., "Love, Law, and Civil Disobedience," in *A Testament of Hope: The Essential Writings and Speeches of Martin Luther King, Jr.*, ed. James M. Washington (New York: HarperCollins, 1986), 52.

60. Robert D. Orr and Susan Salladay, "Wisdom from Health Care," in *Why the Church Needs Bioethics*, ed. John F. Kilner (Grand Rapids, MI: Zondervan, 2011), 216.

61. Hollinger, 265.

62. Tom L. Beauchamp and James F. Childress, *Principles of Biomedical Ethics*, 7th edition (New York: Oxford University Press, 2013), 169. Care must be taken when speaking of treatments that are deemed futile because the literature on this notion and its application in health care is complex and varied. For the qualifications of the concept, see ibid., 169–71.

63. Ibid., 169.

64. Gilbert Meilaender, *Bioethics: A Primer for Christians*, 3rd edition (Grand Rapids, MI: Eerdmans, 2013), 70.

65. John Keown, *Euthanasia, Ethics, and Public Policy: An Argument Against Legalisation* (New York: Cambridge University Press, 2002), 43–44.

66. Ibid., 39.

67. Helga Kuhse, *The Sanctity of Life Doctrine in Medicine: A Critique* (New York: Oxford University Press, 1987), 169.

68. Ibid., 26.

69. Keown, 43.

70. Ibid., 44.

71. Ibid.

72. For a robust Protestant theological account of health and human flourishing, see Neil Messer, *Flourishing: Health, Disease, and Bioethics in Theological Perspective* (Grand Rapids, MI: Eerdmans, 2013).

73. Tony D. Armstrong, "Practicing Compassion for Dying Children," in *Living Well and Dying Faithfully: Christian Practices for End-of-Life Care*, ed. John Swinton and Richard Payne (Grand Rapids, MI: Eerdmans, 2009), 147.

74. Harold A. Carter, *The Prayer Tradition of the Black People* (Valley Forge, PA: Gateway, 1976), 80.

75. Amy Plantinga Pauw, "Dying Well," in *Living Well and Dying Faithfully: Christian Practice for End-of-Life Care*, ed. John Swinton and Richard Payne (Grand Rapids, MI: Eerdmans, 2009), 21.

76. Carter, 95.

77. Patrick T. Smith, "The 'Patient-Family Dyad' as an Interdisciplinary Unit of Hospice Care: Toward an Ethical Justification," in *Hospice Ethics: Policy and Practice in Palliative Care*, ed. Timothy W. Kirk and Bruce Jennings (New York: Oxford University Press, 2014), 144–62.

11

Seventh-Day Adventists and Care for the Newborn

Gerald R. Winslow

A story, like a prism, may open to view nuances otherwise hidden. So, let me begin with a story. Baby Olivia came to the neonatal intensive care unit (NICU) in our medical center nearly three months after her premature birth at twenty-six weeks gestation.[1] By the time I met her, she was six months old. I had been asked by her caregiving team to provide an ethics consultation, a service I have been giving, off and on, for nearly forty years.

Olivia's professional caregivers were conflicted about their plans for her treatment. Some believed they had already done too much. In their view, the suffering caused by medical interventions was far greater than the most likely outcome could possibly warrant. They pointed to some grim facts. Olivia's lungs were compromised. She required a special type of ventilator support with high-tech equipment usually only available in tertiary medical centers. She had already needed numerous episodes of resuscitation. All attempts to wean her from the ventilator had failed, which meant that she could not be transferred to a long-term care facility or to home care. She could only be fed through a gastrostomy tube, and she was growing very slowly. She had also experienced bleeding in her brain—a grade 4 intraventricular hemorrhage with hydrocephaly requiring a shunt. While difficult to predict with precision, Olivia would likely have some degree of intellectual impairment. In the opinion of some members of the caregiving team, it was time to "stop the heroics."

Others saw matters quite differently. When the team met to discuss the options for Olivia's care, one of the senior physicians discussed the fact that she saw no signs of seizures or any evidence of cerebral palsy. She also mentioned the fact that Olivia engaged her caregivers visually. While Olivia remained small, she seemed to be a "fighter" who tolerated the tube feedings fairly well. The lung disease was obviously serious, but another physician cautioned against considering it "end stage." He recalled cases of "kids on vents for two or even three years" who eventually had been weaned successfully. He added, "We are not to the place where we have nothing more to offer." Everyone seemed to agree that

Olivia fared better when one nurse named Angela—a twenty-plus-year veteran of NICU care—was looking after her. It was nurse Angela who was among the strongest advocates for continuing with the current treatment plan and who called attention to the parents' expressed wish to make every medically possible attempt to preserve Olivia's life.

Olivia's parents, both of whom were employed full-time, lived more than two hours away by car. They both indicated that they wanted to be thoroughly involved in decisions about Olivia's care. However, they were seldom able to visit her or speak directly with her nurses and physicians. Despite their difficulties in understanding the details of Olivia's care and the challenges of communicating mostly by telephone, her parents made it entirely clear that they wanted "everything" to be done. They quickly became frustrated or indignant if any questions arose regarding limitations of medical treatment, including an order to stop further attempts at resuscitation. The parents expressed their hope that God would perform a miracle, and they requested the services of a Catholic priest.

Olivia's story raises many questions. Is there one optimal course of action in a case like hers? Who has the final say? What is the best way, if any, to take the parents' religious hope into account? Coming to the primary purpose of this chapter, does it matter at all that the hospital where Olivia received care is operated by Seventh-day Adventists as an expression of their faith?

Before this chapter's conclusion, I will share the outcome of Olivia's story. But I have chosen to open the chapter with her story as a way of framing the context for an account of Adventist[2] beliefs and practices and their relationship to health care for newborn infants. I am an Adventist theologian and ethicist, and I have specialized in biomedical ethics since the 1970s. I work at an Adventist health sciences university that takes as its stated mission "to continue the teaching and healing ministry of Jesus Christ."[3] In a typical year, more than 2,500 babies take their first breaths in one of our facilities. Of course, most of these go home soon after birth, accompanied by joyous parents. If religious faith enters into the hospital experience in any explicit way, it may be through an offer of one of our physicians or nurses to pray with the patient or family, a visit from one of our chaplains, or a response to parents' request for an infant baptism or "baby dedication."

But then there are stories like Olivia's. The NICU where she spent several months has eighty-four licensed beds. While her story has its distinctive features, similar stories occur often. As the only level-1 trauma center for four counties with more than four million inhabitants, and as one of the few tertiary centers for children in Southern California, our hospital must be prepared to provide the highest level of care for newborns with the most complex illnesses and injuries. Adventists have established healthcare institutions of this sort as practical expressions of faith. In this chapter, my goal is to explain some of the Adventist convictions that provide the motivation for engaging in health care and that shape the way that care is given. I will also seek to explain how Adventist beliefs may affect the ways in which Adventists receive health care when it is their turn to be the patients.

The Story of Adventist Health Care

When Adventists first started to offer health care, they could not have imagined what would evolve as the various Adventist health systems today. Under the visionary guidance of early Adventist leader Ellen G. White, Adventists were encouraged to make what was called *health reform* a part of their faithful, personal practice and a part of the Adventist church's service to others.[4] The Western Health Reform Institute was opened in Michigan in September 1866, with Dr. Horatio Lay as its sole physician caring for two patients.[5] Ten years later, the most prominent of early Adventist physicians, Dr. John Harvey Kellogg, became the director.[6]

Under Kellogg's leadership, the institution, renamed the Battle Creek Sanitarium, grew rapidly in size and in public attention.[7] The name *Kellogg* is probably best known in American culture because of the commercial development of breakfast cereals by W. K. Kellogg, younger brother of the physician.[8] The tactic of seeking to change the way Americans ate breakfast was just one illustration of the primary goal of early Adventist health ministry—to encourage healthful living as a way of preventing disease, and to base this commitment on faithfulness to God.[9] The provision of acute care was not an early priority. Adventists often used the word *sanitarium* for their healthcare institutions as a way of signaling the intention to help people regain their health through such natural remedies as clean water, sunlight, a plant-based diet, adequate rest, and regular exercise. The aim of these institutions also included having patients learn about the elements of a lifestyle better suited to preserving health. The plan worked. Over the subsequent decades, people who adopted the health practices advocated by Adventists tended to live longer, healthier lives.[10]

When the Adventist engagement in health care began, much of what passed for medicine was in fact detrimental.[11] Patent remedies, often containing toxic or addictive substances, were widely offered as cures for nearly all ailments. Many medical interventions at the time—such as bloodletting, heroin for the common cold, and radium for arthritis and diabetes—caused far more harm than good. Perhaps because of my surname, one of the illustrations I find most memorable is Mrs. Winslow's Soothing Syrup. The formula contained alcohol, morphine, and opium, and it was advertised as the perfect medicine for teething children.[12] An 1861 edition of the *New York Times* carried the glowing testimonials of satisfied customers, and added the fact that millions of bottles had been sold. The remarkable price was twenty-five cents![13] It was not until 1906 that this patent remedy was banned by the US government. In many ways, the Adventist rejection of patent drugs, as well as abstinence from tobacco products and alcoholic beverages, represented counter-cultural expressions of a faith that included a commitment to human health. The same was true of the Adventist promotion of natural remedies and a vegetarian diet. The idea was to keep people healthy and out of acute care hospitals. The building and operation of such hospitals came later.

What were the factors that led a small American religious denomination, dedicated to establishing sanitariums for regaining and maintaining health, to build many modern hospitals, nursing homes, clinics, and even health sciences universities around the world? First, scientifically credible, evidence-based health care emerged with increasingly noteworthy success. Over the same decades, Adventist institutions provided accredited education to thousands of healthcare professionals, including nurses, physicians, dentists, and public health experts. So, when the efforts at health promotion and disease prevention failed, as all of them eventually do, Adventists recognized the increasing value of providing acute care in hospitals dedicated to serving the needs of the whole person, including needs for spiritually nurturing care. The move away from the language and culture of sanitariums, with their long patient stays, toward acute care hospitals occasioned some Adventist soul-searching.[14] However, the wisdom of adopting the best prevailing medical practices won out, and hospitals capable of caring for patients like Olivia became part of the health ministry of Adventists. At their best, such acute care hospitals have sought to preserve the essential principles on which that ministry was founded while also incorporating thoroughly evidence-based acute care medicine.

Beliefs Informing Adventist Care

At present, Adventists officially list twenty-eight "fundamental beliefs."[15] Most of these are held in common with other Christian denominations, and many of the beliefs are also shared with the other monotheistic religions of the world. For the purposes of this chapter, I will call on four Adventist convictions that significantly inform Adventist reasons for engaging in health care and also shape the way care is provided.

Creation

Much about Adventist faith and practice is molded by an abiding belief in the providential creation of the world. Adventists believe that the all-wise and gracious Maker of Heaven and Earth intended for human beings to live in peace with each other, with their environment, and with God. Humans were given the responsibility, as faithful stewards, to care for the creation.[16] Adventists also accept the creation Sabbath, made holy by God, as a blessed gift to humans.[17] It serves as a perpetual reminder of the Creator's power and goodness, while also providing needed rest not only for human beings but also for the animals to which human beings relate.[18] Even the Adventist emphasis on a plant-based diet is founded, in part, on the belief that the ideal diet for human beings is described in the Genesis account of creation.[19]

In terms of the way it affects the Adventist commitment to health care, one of the most significant beliefs, stemming from the creation story, is that human beings are created in the "image of God."[20] Adventists understand this to mean that human life is a sacred gift from God, and life deserves to be protected. It also means that every human being is given dignity that calls for respect, regardless of any assessments of individual excellence or merit. Each human life, no matter how flawed or fragile it may appear, is graced by divinely appointed nobility. This conviction should have obvious implications for the care of patients like baby Olivia. Notwithstanding her difficult start in life and her guarded prognosis, she is deserving of loving care. Indeed, her very vulnerability should elicit powerful commitments to serve her best interests as one who is a beloved child of God.

Human Wholeness

The Adventist belief in creation also has implications for an understanding of human wholeness. Adventists believe that, by the Creator's design, each person is a spiritual and physical *unity*. Adventists fundamentally believe that every human being "is an indivisible unity of body, mind, and spirit, dependent upon God for life and breath. . . ."[21] Adventists reject body-soul *dualism*—the notion that an immortal soul comes to inhabit the physical reality of the body. From the perspective of Adventist anthropology, it is correct to say that a person *is* a soul and not that a person *has* a soul. For Adventists, this is not just a conceptual or linguistic nicety. The belief in human wholeness is fundamentally important for why and how Adventists provide health care. The goal of such care is to restore, to the extent possible, human wholeness in which all dimensions of life are unified through connection to a spiritually meaningful core. Health care that focuses only on the physical well-being of the person fails to serve the larger goal of human wholeness. In cases like baby Olivia's, it is not just her wholeness that is sought; it is also the wholeness of her parents and the wholeness of her caregivers. Faith-inspired, spiritually nurturing health care, as understood by

Adventists, is founded on the reality that God created human beings as spiritually attuned whole persons.

Spiritual Commitment to Health

The Adventist understanding of human wholeness leads to a spiritual commitment to preserve and promote human health. In recent decades, there has been a growing interest in the relationship of religious practices, spirituality, and health outcomes. There is widespread recognition of the positive relationship between human spirituality and human health.[22] Most of the attention has been given to the potential benefits to physical health that stem from various religious or spiritual practices. Far less notice has been given to the prospects of more vibrant spiritual life made possible through better health practices. The Adventist view of wholeness encompasses both: the spiritual benefits of preserving health, and the health benefits of vibrant spirituality. In this regard, an important biblical passage for Adventists is the Christian apostle Paul's admonition to believers: "do you not know that your body is a temple of the Holy Spirit within you, which you have from God, and that you are not your own? For you were bought with a price; therefore glorify God in your body."[23]

The belief that healthful living is a spiritual responsibility has led Adventists to renounce destructive habits such as the use of tobacco and the abuse and drugs and alcohol. This same belief has also given impetus to adopt a plant-based diet and promote environmental efforts for clean air and pure water. Adventists believe they have a God-given mandate to share information about healthful living and encourage the adoption of a healthy lifestyle. So much of what eventually leads to the necessity of acute medical care could be prevented if people understood and were empowered to follow better health principles. Adventists are eager to ensure that these principles are available to all.

Worldwide Mission

A founding example for Adventist health care comes from Jesus' instruction to his disciples: "Then Jesus called the twelve together and gave them power and authority over all demons and to cure diseases, and he sent them out to proclaim the kingdom of God and to heal. . . . They departed and went through the villages, bringing the good news and curing diseases everywhere."[24] Adventists believe that their distinctive calling entails prophetic outreach to the entire planet. They are not content to limit their health ministry to a particular nation or a region of the world. The commitment to a worldwide mission has led to the establishment of some form of Adventist health ministry in nearly 200 countries. At present, this work is conducted in 947 different languages.[25] As someone commented recently, "At the end of nearly every bad road there seems to be an Adventist health facility." While that is surely an exaggeration, the goal of Adventists is to make spiritually enriching health principles and health care available to every human being on earth.

To accomplish this enormous task, Adventists have needed to establish schools that could prepare students for such service. Currently, the denomination operates 7,579 schools with more than 85,000 teachers. Wherever Adventism has succeeded most fully in accomplishing its mission, there are usually at least three synergistic institutions: a church, a school, and a health facility.

It is important to add that the services provided by Adventist schools and healthcare institutions are intended to be available to all members of the community, regardless of their religious affiliation, or lack thereof, and regardless of any other social distinctions. Adventists believe that the combination of excellent education and excellent health care will help to establish the well-being of whole communities. Evidence from decades of experience in many cultural environments has supported the wisdom of this combination of faith-based services. The success of these endeavors is, as Adventists see it, a result of God's guidance.

Beliefs Informing Adventists' Reception of Care

In addition to the Adventist core beliefs just described, there are nuances of those convictions and their corresponding practices that may affect the way Adventists receive care when they or their family members are patients. Healthcare professionals who are caring for Adventists could benefit from considering the practical implications of five such beliefs described later.

Commitment to Healthful Living

Adventists will typically value a caregiving environment that respects their commitment to live healthfully, in an atmosphere as free as possible from factors that are deleterious to human health. For example, Adventists will value a tobacco-free setting in which they are not subjected to second-hand or even what is now called *third-hand* exposure to residues of tobacco or its primary drug, nicotine.[26] In practical terms, this means avoiding surroundings that have the obvious odor of tobacco, or also the pollutants released by e-cigarettes. Similarly, Adventists will appreciate an environment that excludes the use of alcoholic beverages. Many Adventists also avoid the use of coffee or caffeinated drinks.

A significant percentage of Adventists follow the advice to choose a vegetarian diet. This is not a requirement of Adventist membership, but it is given as counsel regarding the ideal diet. Thus, many Adventists will appreciate meatless, plant-based dietary options. Those Adventists who are not vegetarians will avoid pork and shellfish.

Most Adventists will welcome health education as part of receiving health care, especially if the education includes attention to elements of a healthy life-style likely to be of benefit in their situation. Information about natural remedies, such as exercise and dietary changes that may enhance the chances of healing, are likely to be valued.

While none of these factors regarding healthful living might seem directly applicable to the care of the newborn, they are apt to affect the way Adventist family members relate to the care environment.

Belief in Providential Care

Adventists believe in divine guidance through the work of the Holy Spirit and in the power of the Creator to aid in the healing processes. This belief includes an emphasis on the importance of prayer. Adventists take seriously these words of Scripture: "The prayer of faith will save the sick, and the Lord will raise them up."[27] And "Rejoice in hope, be patient in suffering, persevere in prayer."[28] Thus, most Adventist patients, or their families, will appreciate sincere offers of prayer from caregivers. Adventists are, of course, aware of the fact that God's answers to prayer do not always lead to the hoped-for outcome. They are also thoroughly committed to health care based on scientific evidence. At the same time, they will draw strength and comfort from authentic attention to providential presence and power.

Some Adventist patients or family members may also wish to pray for their caregivers. If such offers can be accepted in good faith, Adventists are likely to be grateful for the opportunity to pray with and for their caregivers.

The Adventist perspective on providential care can best be described as personal cooperation with the power of God. At their best, Adventists take responsibility for their own efforts to collaborate with the will of the Creator. As one of the founders of the Adventist health ministry commented, "To make God's grace our own, we must act our part. His grace is given to work in us to will and to do, but never as a substitute for our effort."[29] In the context of health care, the practical effect of this belief is the willingness to be engaged in collaboration with God's will in the restoration of health, combining the best of scientific medicine with spiritually nurturing care.

Honoring Sacred Time

As the name *Seventh-day Adventist* signifies, Adventists are Sabbatarian—they believe in the sacredness of the seventh day (or Saturday) Sabbath, which they observe from sunset on Friday evening until sunset on Saturday evening. During the hours of the Sabbath, Adventists seek to refrain from ordinary work in order to devote time to prayer, bible study, religious services, and acts of compassion for those in need. The Sabbath is a time when Adventists find restoration of personal wholeness and the wholeness of the faith community.

The commitment to Sabbath sacredness does not mean, however, that Adventists cease providing or receiving health care on the seventh day of the week. Following the example of Jesus, who healed the sick on Sabbath,[30] Adventists take responsibility for health and healing every day of the week.

For Adventists who are receiving health care, any acknowledgement on the part of caregivers that they understand the significance that this sacred time has for Adventists is likely to be warmly appreciated. Offers to pray with Adventist patients or their families during the Sabbath hours, for example, would likely be a particularly helpful blessing.

Freedom of Conscience

Adventists place a high value on respect for personal conscience, with a special concern for the preservation of religious liberty. Since 1906, Adventists have published a journal simply titled *Liberty* that is devoted to promoting freedom of conscience around the world.[31] The Adventist church sees itself as having a prophetic calling to champion the human right to practice one's faith and follow one's own conscientious convictions. This has led the church to support the religious liberty of socially marginalized groups, even when the views and practices of such groups differ widely from those of Adventists.[32]

This belief in personal conscience has had significant implications for Adventist bioethics. For example, except in rare instances, such as serious risks to the life of the pregnant woman, Adventists affirm the duty to protect prenatal life. But the Adventist guidelines on abortion also make it clear that the final decision about continuing a pregnancy belongs to the one who is pregnant, and the guidelines include these words: "any attempts to coerce women either to remain pregnant or to terminate pregnancy should be rejected as infringements of personal freedom."[33] Later in this chapter, the same kind of commitment to individual conscience will be in evidence in Adventists' ethical guidance for care at the end of life.

One noteworthy implication of the belief in personal liberty is that Adventists do not practice infant baptism. They believe that a child should mature in her or his own spiritual convictions such that a thoughtful decision to accept or reject religious faith can be made. However, some Adventists may request that their infant have a dedication service in which prayer is offered for the infant and his or her parents.

With reference to care in the NICU, the significance of the Adventist commitment to personal freedom of conscience means that Adventists seek to respect the religious convictions of those who are receiving care. For example, when the parents of baby Olivia request the religious services of a priest or want to pray for a miracle for their baby, Adventist caregivers should respond with respect for such desires. And when Adventists are the recipients of care, they will expect to receive the same regard for their distinctive religious convictions.

Hope for Eternal Life

As with all Christians, Adventists accept the promise that faith in Jesus will lead to eternal life: "For God so loved the world that he gave his only Son, so that everyone who believes in him may not perish but may have eternal life."[34] This hope for spending eternity with God and with the believer's loved ones can be a source of great comfort when persons are facing serious medical diagnoses. Adventist families whose infants are receiving care in the NICU will likely be heartened by sharing this faith.

When death occurs, Adventists believe that the deceased person enters into a time of rest, awaiting the resurrection and eternal life. Because of their firm belief in body and soul unity, Adventists do *not* believe that a conscious soul, disconnected from the body, goes directly to heaven immediately after the death of the body. In the words of Adventists' statement of *Fundamental Beliefs*, "God, who alone is immortal, will grant eternal life to His redeemed. Until that day death is an unconscious state for all people."[35] Adventists believe that God will raise those who have died in faith to a wonderfully restored existence in God's presence forever. Here is an example of a scriptural passage from St. Paul that gives believers such hope: "Brothers and sisters, we do not want you to be uninformed about those who sleep in death, so that you do not grieve like the rest of mankind, who have no hope. For we believe that Jesus died and rose again, and so we believe that God will bring with Jesus those who have fallen asleep in him."[36]

One practical implication of the Adventist belief about death, when it comes to the loss of a newborn's life, is that mention of hope for the resurrection is likely to be comforting. However, it is not helpful to suggest to Adventists that a deceased loved one is now looking down from heaven. Also unhelpful would be words similar to those I heard once from a healthcare professional with good intentions but poor information. She sought to comfort the parents, whose newborn had just died, by explaining that God needed another "angel to help out in Heaven." Silence and the practice of being compassionately present, as one who understands grief, would be far better at such times.

Care at the End of Life

One way to give additional insight into how Adventists both give and receive health care is to share the seven principles Adventists officially espouse for care at the end of life. Elaboration of these principles offers the opportunity to understand more fully some of the central values that inform Adventist caregiving and receiving.[37] The principles are also likely to have implications for care in the NICU.

Veracity

The first principle in the Adventist consensus statement regarding care at life's end calls for telling patients, or their responsible family members, the truth. The statement says, "A person who is approaching the end of life, and is capable of understanding, deserves to know the truth about his or her condition, the treatment choices, and the possible outcomes."[38] In the treatment of newborn infants, of course, this means sharing accurate information with whomever has accepted family responsibility for the baby. The statement adds that "the truth should not be withheld but shared with Christian love and with sensitivity to the patient's personal and cultural circumstances."

The commitment to give truthful information about diagnoses, prognoses, and alternatives for treatment has grown in American culture during my lifetime. I can easily remember attitudes of healthcare professionals in the 1950s and 1960s when it was much less common to convey complete and accurate information, especially when the news was bad. It was not unusual to withhold information on the grounds that it would be discouraging or even terrifying for the patient or family members. Times have changed. The responsibility for giving people the essential facts, as best they can be known, is now taught to healthcare professional students, included in the professional codes of conduct, and reinforced by legal requirements. Still, in the richly multicultural setting I know best, it is not uncommon to encounter divergent attitudes about the commitment to full disclosure of the medical condition and treatment options. The Adventist statement acknowledges such cultural differences and calls for sensitivity regarding how best to share the truth. But the statement also makes it clear that there is a solemn responsibility to be compassionately truthful.

With reference to treatment of newborns, the practical effect of this principle would lead caregivers to be as forthcoming with the truth as the babies' parents or guardians can understand. My observation is that discovery of the best ways to share such information occurs over time through the example of experienced, artful caregivers and through sometimes difficult experiences.

Freedom

As mentioned earlier in this chapter, Adventists are committed to a high level of respect for personal conscience. So it is not surprising that this value is included in the consensus statement on care for those who are dying with these words: "After seeking divine guidance and considering the interests of those affected by the decision as well as medical advice, a person who is capable of deciding should determine whether to accept or reject life-extending medical interventions. Such persons should not be forced to submit to medical treatment that they find unacceptable."[39]

Such a sweeping statement could obviously raise significant questions in a NICU, where inevitably the decisions to start, continue, or stop life-extending care are being made for the patient by others, usually the parents in consultation with healthcare professionals. As the story of baby Olivia illustrates, there are times when the professional caregivers do not agree fully on the goals of treatment, especially when it comes to decisions about withdrawal of life-extending interventions. Nothing in the Adventist statement of principles will ensure easy resolution of the perennial questions about ethics in the NICU—questions that have been described, analyzed, and debated now for decades.[40] For example, within Adventist hospitals that provide specialized care for newborn infants, cases may occur in which parents refuse some medical intervention that doctors believe is essential for saving an infant's life. If the matter cannot be resolved, and if proceeding with the treatment requires an immediate court order, such legal oversight may be deemed necessary. Of course, the earnest hope is that some combination of careful discussion on the part of caregivers with the family, possibly an ethics consultation, and the availability of a multidisciplinary professional team, including such services as those of a medical social worker and a chaplain, will facilitate a harmonious resolution. The Adventist respect for the autonomy of parents does not entirely eliminate rare situations requiring a court decision. The principle should incline caregivers, however, to give thorough and respectful consideration to the parents' perspective.

Family

Adventists affirm the value of nurturing relationships within the context of a family and a community of faith. In caring for persons as they approach the end of life, these relationships can be especially important. In the words of the Adventist consensus statement, "Decisions about human life are best made within the context of healthy family relationships after considering medical advice. . . . Except in extraordinary circumstances, medical or legal professionals should defer decisions about medical interventions for a dying person to those closest to that individual."[41] In decisions about the care of the newborn, the application of this norm would call for the full engagement of both parents if they are willing to participate in the process. Nothing in the Adventist statement of principles would lead to favoring one parent over the other in making the required medical choices.

Most of the time, this is the arrangement that works best. Even with the stress of serious medical diagnoses, most families are able to find the necessary resilience to collaborate with attending physicians in arriving at mutually agreeable decisions. Among the sad exceptions are those times when the patient is unrepresented by any family member, as sometimes happens even with those newly born. In such rare cases, the influence of the principle of family solidarity would lead caregivers to genuine diligence in seeking to find and connect with caring family members. If such efforts fail, ethical intuitions and legal opinions about the value of having a court-appointed guardian are likely to differ. In my view, decisions about the goals of treatment and the most appropriate means for achieving those goals are best kept as close as possible to the setting in which the care is given. Safeguards can be put in place with the intention of ensuring that the best interests of the newborn take priority.

Limitations

The Adventist consensus on end-of-life care includes the frank acknowledgement that there are times when it is ethically permissible to forgo life-extending medical interventions. For example, the statement says, "when medical care merely preserves bodily functions, without hope of returning a patient to mental awareness, it is futile and may, in good conscience, be withheld or withdrawn." The statement also indicates that "life-extending medical treatments may be omitted or stopped if they only add to the patient's suffering or needlessly prolong the process of dying."[42]

The practical consequence of these words for Adventist caregivers and care receivers is that it is ethically responsible to assess whether or not medical interventions make sense in light of the patient's condition, the hoped-for benefits, and burdens of the treatments. Adventists are not committed to extending life at all costs, regardless of whether or not the probability of medical success would justify the burdens of the medical measures.

Prohibition of Killing

Adventists officially forswear the practice of intentionally ending the life of any patient. The consensus statement avers that "Seventh-day Adventists do not practice 'mercy killing' or assist in suicide. They are opposed to active euthanasia, the intentional taking of the life of a suffering or dying person."[43] For those who see no ethically relevant difference between withdrawing artificial life support and taking measures directly intended to end human life, the Adventist statement may seem incoherent. However, Adventists make what they consider to be a crucial distinction between stopping medical treatments that are deemed useless or harmful and actions intended to kill the patient. In previous decades, this distinction would need little explanation. But as more and more jurisdictions are moving to authorize medically assisted suicide, there seems to be greater need to justify insisting on the ethically important difference between ceasing efforts to hold off death caused by illness and actions designed to end the life of a person who is suffering. All indications are that Adventists will continue to hold to this distinction and shape their practices accordingly.

The prohibition regarding intentionally ending the life of a patient will not alter the usual practice of medicine in an American NICU. The prospect of active euthanasia for infants is not only morally abhorrent to most people, it is also illegal in all US jurisdictions. However, the prohibition is ethically significant for a number of reasons. It reminds caregivers that the gift of human life is sacred and deserving of protection, with special care given to our most vulnerable members of society. It helps to establish safeguards intended to make sure that decisions to stop medically ineffective or inappropriate care do not slide gradually toward actions that intentionally cause death. Finally, for people of faith, the prohibition serves as a counsel of humility, reminding us that we are not the Creator of human life, and we are not authorized to extinguish human life.

Alleviation of Suffering

In the official statement on care for the dying, Adventists have affirmed the moral importance of alleviating human suffering. After citing the well-known story of the *Good Samaritan*,[44] the statement says, "It is a Christian responsibility to relieve pain and suffering to the fullest extent possible, not to include active euthanasia."[45] The document specifically rejects attempts to valorize pain, as if pain could earn merit for the one who suffers. Instead, affirmation is given to the ethical wisdom of making comfort the primary goal of medical care when it is clear that curative goals cannot be achieved.

One practical consequence of this principle in all of health care, including the NICU, is to emphasize the importance of highly skilled comfort care, especially in situations when the patient is dying. The fact that the newborn cannot tell caregivers about her or his discomfort makes it all the more important to be attentive to the signs of suffering and to seek ways that will bring relief and comfort.

It should be acknowledged that there are times when the condition of a newborn makes it uncertain whether or not continued medical interventions are at all likely to achieve their desired goals. Baby Olivia's story was just such a case. Some caregivers thought that the primary goal should shift to comfort care. Others disagreed. There are some conditions, different from Olivia's, for which the consensus of caregivers has usually favored comfort care, without attempts to extend life. Anencephaly is typically considered to be one example. The life of an anencephalic infant is usually only a few hours to a few days in length, and the standard approach of caregivers is respectfully providing comfort care. There are other conditions, however, such as Trisomy 13 and Trisomy 18, for which consensus is less obvious, and traditional approaches favoring comfort care and disfavoring life-extending care are under reconsideration. The Adventist principles do not provide specific guidance for a list of various conditions. Rather, Adventist convictions would tend to favor giving significant weight to the decisions of parents, or other authorized decision makers, based on the best evidence regarding medical prognoses and in consultation with medical experts.

Justice

The final principle in the Adventist statement expresses a commitment to human equality and fairness. In the words of the statement, "The biblical principle of justice prescribes that added care be given the needs of those who are defenseless and dependent. . . . Because of their vulnerable condition, special care should be taken to ensure that dying persons are treated with respect for their dignity and without unfair discrimination." The statement adds words of caution against basing care "on perceptions of [patients'] social worthiness."[46]

It would be difficult to imagine any patient more vulnerable than a premature infant receiving care in a NICU. The biblical sense of justice, on which the Adventist statement relies, is fundamentally committed to giving strategic priority to the care of such vulnerable members of our community. Passages like this one from Isaiah make this point: "Learn to do good; seek justice, rescue the oppressed, defend the orphan, plead for the widow."[47]

One practical implication of the commitment to justice is the willingness to challenge conventional customs that lead to many types of discrimination. For example, as a worldwide religious movement, Adventism lives in cultures that may traditionally disfavor a particular racial group or one of the sexes or some religious minority. Because unfair discrimination is often so deeply entrenched, so common, and so destructive of the dignity Adventists believe the Creator intends for all members of the human family, the Adventist church has made clear statements against such discrimination and in favor of human equality: "In Christ we are a new creation; distinctions of race, culture, learning, and nationality, and differences between high and low, rich and poor, male and female, must not be divisive among us. We are all equal in Christ. . . ."[48] Real-life applications of this principle of equality would obviously prohibit discrimination in the care of newborns based on their sex, race, religion, nationality, or any other morally irrelevant criteria.

It would be misleading to suggest that the principle of justice has been fully effective in any culture known to me. The society with which I am most familiar still has much to learn about the depths of this prophetic message of justice. Adventists are committed to helping create and sustain healthcare institutions that treat all persons fairly.

Conclusion

The context of the NICU, in a religiously and culturally pluralistic society, often provides vivid opportunities to test the application of deeply held convictions. The story of baby Olivia, with which I began this chapter, was such a test. The healthcare professionals attending to Olivia found themselves with divergent views about the best path forward. The parents were insistent that their beliefs about what was best for Olivia be respected. Despite differing perceptions regarding the most appropriate ways to care for her, there was never disagreement that the primary goal of our care was to do what was best for Olivia.

Over the three months that followed my first encounter with Olivia, her condition continued to worsen. It became increasingly evident that Olivia's lungs were too compromised, and multiple other factors were converging to make her survival impossible. Finally, with the help of their priest and the support of compassionate caregivers, the parents concluded that the goals of Olivia's care should focus primarily on her comfort. The healthcare professionals, who had invested so much in keeping Olivia alive, agreed with the parents. Artificial life support was withdrawn, and at the age of nine months, Olivia died.

Did we try too hard or too long? Could we have arrived at the same conclusion months earlier? No ethically sensitive person can fully avoid the discomfort of such questions. Hospitals often feel like spaces in which this kind of discomfort and the uncertainties associated with human suffering are concentrated. As Olivia's case illustrates, there are circumstances in which even our best efforts, our most sophisticated medical technology, and our best ethical deliberations seem insufficient.

At the same time, hospitals are places in which the courage, grace, and resilience of caring persons are on full display. This is often especially true in the NICU. The resources of religious faith have the potential to sustain the kind of care that is not only medically excellent but also spiritually nurturing. Along with many other communities of faith, Adventists have accepted the extraordinary responsibility of creating and operating healthcare institutions that seek to provide such care, and to do so with ethical integrity. Most of the time, the care of newborns offered by Adventists, or received by Adventists, will be just what would be expected at any evidence-based and ethically sensitive NICU in societies with highly advanced healthcare systems. The effects of deeply held religious convictions will seldom, if ever, be directly observable in the specific interventions at any given moment. Still, the beliefs will be at work in shaping of character traits and in development of the motivations for action. At their best, faith-inspired hospitals and the professional caregivers who work in them can draw on powerful assets of the spirit that foster compassion and respect for every patient and family member for whom care is essential.

In this chapter, I have sought to describe some of the more salient Adventist beliefs that have inspired a relatively small Christian denomination to make immense investments in state-of-the-art medical care, including neonatal intensive care. My hope is that this explanation of Adventists' faith will help readers toward a clearer understanding of why and how Adventists provide care that is scientifically sound and spiritually empowering. At the same time, I hope that healthcare professionals, regardless of their own religious background or lack thereof, will have gained some insights into how best to serve those who are members of the Adventist community of faith.

Notes

1. The details of this account have been altered to ensure protection of confidential, personal information.
2. Throughout this chapter, I use *Adventist* and *Adventism* to refer to the Christian denomination whose full name is Seventh-day Adventist.

3. Information about Loma Linda University Health, including the mission statement, is available at http://medical-center.lomalindahealth.org/about-us (accessed August 15, 2017).

4. The best scholarly account of Ellen White's influence on health—both within Adventism and the larger culture—is Ronald L. Numbers, *Prophetess of Health: A Study of Ellen G. White* (Grand Rapids, MI: Eerdmans, 2008). For White's most influential work on the subject, see Ellen G. White, *The Ministry of Healing* (Mountain View, CA: Pacific Press, 1909). For a recent collection of scholarly essays on White's historical and cultural significance, see Terrie Dopp Aamodt, Gary Land, and Ronald L. Numbers, ed., *Ellen Harmon White: American Prophet* (New York: Oxford University Press, 2014).

5. The story of the Western Health Reform Institute is told briefly at http://www. heritagebattlecreek.org/index.php?option=com_content&view=article&id=95 &Itemid=73 (accessed August 16, 2017). More information about the Institute is also available at https://en.wikipedia.org/wiki/Battle_Creek_Sanitarium (accessed August 16, 2017).

6. A repository of John Harvey Kellogg's papers is maintained by Michigan State University and is described, with a short biography of Kellogg, at http://archives. msu.edu/findaid/013.html (accessed August 16, 2017).

7. The story of Battle Creek Sanitarium is widely available; a brief account may be found at http://ellenwhite.org/content/location/battle-creek-sanitarium-battle-creek-michigan-us (accessed August 16, 2017).

8. The story of W. K. Kellogg is nicely told at https://www.wkkf.org/who-we-are/ history-legacy (accessed August 16, 2017).

9. Brian C. Wilson, *Dr. John Harvey Kellogg and the Religion of Biologic Living* (Bloomington, IN: Indiana University Press, 2014). Wilson provides a fascinating history of Kellogg's rise to prominence as a physician and innovator, his connection of religion to healthful living, and his eventual enthusiasm for eugenics.

10. For a comprehensive review of outcomes related to Adventist health practices, see Gary E. Fraser, *Diet, Life Expectancy and Chronic Disease: Studies of Seventh-Day Adventists and Other Vegetarians* (New York: Oxford University Press, 2003).

11. For a colorful account of nineteenth-century patent medicine and dubious medical interventions, see Otto Bettmann, *The Good Old Days: They Were Terrible!* (New York: Random House, 1974).

12. A photo of the bottle label for Mrs. Winslow's Soothing Syrup and a listing of some of the ingredients can be found at https://en.wikipedia.org/wiki/Mrs._Winslow%27s_ Soothing_Syrup (accessed June 9, 2019). For the record, the Mrs. Winslow of soothing syrup fame was not the mother of this chapter's author.

13. The *New York Times* copy can be seen at https://timesmachine.nytimes.com/timesm achine/1861/09/19/90548122.html?action=click&contentCollection=Archives&mo dule=LedeAsset&region=ArchiveBody&pgtype=article&pageNumber=5 (accessed June 9, 2019).

14. Ronald A. Bettle, "Is the Sanitarium Obsolete?," *Ministry: International Journal for Pastors* 44 (March 1971).

15. General Conference of Seventh-day Adventists, "Fundamental Beliefs," accessed August 27, 2017, https://www.adventist.org/fileadmin/adventist.org/files/articles/official-statements/28Beliefs-Web.pdf.

16. Genesis 2:15, NRSV, "The LORD God took the man and put him in the garden of Eden to till it and keep it."

17. Genesis 2:3, NRSV, "God blessed the seventh day and hallowed it, because on it God rested from all the work that he had done in creation." See also Exodus 20:8–11.

18. Exodus 20:8–11.

19. Genesis 1:29, NRSV, "God said, 'See, I have given you every plant yielding seed that is upon the face of all the earth, and every tree with seed in its fruit; you shall have them for food.'"

20. Genesis 1:27, NRSV, "So God created humankind in his image, in the image of God he created them; male and female he created them."

21. General Conference of Seventh-day Adventists, "Fundamental Beliefs," last modified 2015, accessed August 27, 2017, https://www.adventist.org/fileadmin/adventist.org/files/articles/official-statements/28Beliefs-Web.pdf.

22. See, e.g., Harold G. Koenig, Dana E. King, and Verna Benner Carson, *Handbook of Religion and Health*, 2nd edition (New York: Oxford University Press, 2012).

23. I Corinthians 6:19–20, NRSV.

24. Luke 9:1–2, 4, NRSV.

25. Statistics about Adventist health and educational ministries are available at https://www.adventist.org/en/information/statistics/ (last updated 2015; accessed August 27, 2017).

26. See, for example, J. Taylor Hays, "What Is Third-Hand Smoke, and Why Is It a Concern?" *Mayo Clinic*, accessed September 16, 2017, http://www.mayoclinic.org/healthy-lifestyle/adult-health/expert-answers/third-hand-smoke/faq-20057791.

27. James 5:15, NRSV.

28. Romans 12:12, NRSV.

29. Ellen G. White, *From Splendor to Shadow* (Mountain View, CA: Pacific Press, 1986), 252.

30. John 5:1–17.

31. Editions of *Liberty* may be viewed at http://libertymagazine.org/ (accessed September 16, 2017).

32. Gerald R. Winslow, "A Prophetic Minority: Reflections on Adventist Social Ethics," in *Journeys to Wisdom: Festchrift in Honour of Michael Pearson*, ed. Andreas Bochmann, Manuela Casti Yeagley, and Jean-Claude Verrecchia (Bracknell, UK: Newbold, 2015), 133–51.

33. General Conference of Seventh-day Adventists, "Guidelines on Abortion," adopted October 12, 1992; accessed September 16, 2017, https://www.adventist.org/en/information/official-statements/guidelines/article/go/0/abortion/.

34. John 3:16, NRSV.

35. General Conference of Seventh-day Adventists, "Fundamental Beliefs," last modified 2015, accessed September 23, 2017, https://www.adventist.org/fileadmin/adventist.org/files/articles/official-statements/28Beliefs-Web.pdf.

36. 1 Thessalonians 4:13–14, NIV.
37. The Adventist principles for end-of-life care are found in General Conference of Seventh-day Adventists, "A Statement of Consensus on Care for the Dying," last modified October 1992, accessed September 23, 2017, https://news.adventist.org/en/all-news/news/go/1998-03-30/a-statement-of-consensus-on-care-for-the-dying/.
38. Ibid.
39. Ibid.
40. See, e.g., this comprehensive book from the 1980s: Earl E. Shelp, *Born to Die? Deciding the Fate of Critically Ill Newborns* (New York: The Free Press, 1986).
41. General Conference of Seventh-day Adventists, "A Statement of Consensus on Care for the Dying," last modified October 1992, accessed September 23, 2017, https://news.adventist.org/en/all-news/news/go/1998-03-30/a-statement-of-consensus-on-care-for-the-dying/.
42. Ibid.
43. Ibid.
44. Luke 10:25–37.
45. General Conference of Seventh-day Adventists, "A Statement of Consensus on Care for the Dying," last modified October 1992, accessed September 23, 2017, https://news.adventist.org/en/all-news/news/go/1998-03-30/a-statement-of-consensus-on-care-for-the-dying/.
46. Ibid.
47. Isaiah 1:17 (NRSV).
48. General Conference of Seventh-day Adventists, "Fundamental Beliefs," last modified 2015, accessed November 5, 2017, https://www.adventist.org/en/beliefs/church/unity-in-the-body-of-christ/.

Afterword

Vincent C. Smith

I am an African American neonatologist who has worked in a neonatal intensive care unit (NICU) for the past twenty years. I am not now nor have I ever been the parent of a preterm infant. All the experiences that I relate and the perspective that I bring are from the point of view of a physician. In this chapter, I was asked to explain from my personal point of view how I feel that religious and spiritual belief systems are involved in providing critical and end-of-life care in the NICU. Rather than focusing on the available literature written on the topic, this chapter represents reflections of a provider who works in this area daily. The thoughts, opinions, and musings shared here are from one person's perspective and are not necessarily representative or reflective of any particular group.

With that in mind, I will begin reviewing the guiding tenets (i.e., religion, faith, doctrine, and spirituality) for this discussion. These tenets can have overlapping aspects, in addition to their unique features. For clarity of discussion, I will provide some definitions to make sure we are using common terminology. *Religion* refers to the belief in or worship of a superhuman controlling power, which many think of in terms of a personal God or gods. I view religion as a set of beliefs and practices that are shared by a group. My view of religion involves some sort of "holy" teaching that typically involves a religious leader who holds some sway over the followers of the religion. *Faith* is a strong belief in God or in the principles of religion based on spiritual apprehension rather than proof. Faith is a series of beliefs that can be applied to a given circumstance or situation as an individual deems appropriate. Unlike religion, faith does not have to involve any particular group or practice. *Doctrine* implies a creed or credo held and taught by a church, political party, or other group. Doctrine is similar to a list of rules that one follows. Doctrines have flexibility in that they can be associated with religion, faith, or spirituality as an individual deems necessary. *Spirituality* signifies the quality of being concerned with the human spirit or soul as opposed to material or physical things. I view spirituality as a belief in some form of higher power or order in the universe.

Although I believe there are distinct differences between religion, faith, doctrine, and spirituality, that is not the point of this discussion. It would be very easy to get lost in semantics. To avoid this, I am going to use the all-encompassing term *belief systems* to cover all the aspects of religion, faith, doctrine, and spirituality collectively. In this context, belief systems will replace the individual terms.

In this chapter, I will attempt to describe what I consider to be some salient points about being a provider in the NICU and the role that a family's belief system plays in critical and end-of-life care for their newborn. I have divided the chapter into the following sections:

- My Understanding of the Role of Belief Systems
- The Contextual Framework of My Personal Belief System
- How I Perceive that Belief Systems Affect NICU Families
- What I Have Learned from Others about Specific Belief Systems
- Why I Have Come to Believe in the Power of Belief Systems

My Understanding of the Role of Belief Systems

Belief systems serve an important role in society. They can provide familiarity in the form of ritual, community, heritage, and culture. They can provide comfort in troubling times. They can help one endure hardships. They can allow one to remain optimistic in the absence of reassurance. Arguably, one of the most important roles that belief systems play is to help individuals manage a crisis.

If life consisted solely of joy and happiness, it is questionable how necessary having a belief system would be. Given that in every life, there are challenges and times of stress and strife, it is belief systems that aid individuals with coping. This is especially true during times of suffering when people feel the most powerless and vulnerable. During times like these, it is can be hard to understand why the crisis is occurring and what can be done to quell it. In fact, the answer is often not known or knowable. In that situation, it would be easy to get depressed and give up. It is during these times that a belief system can help one endure.

One situation in which people often feel powerless and are in crisis mode is when they have a loved one in the NICU. For many families, having a baby that needs NICU care is the worst thing that has ever happened to them. It is often during these times that belief systems become much more actively relevant.

The Contextual Framework of My Personal Belief System

It is rare that during my performance of my job that I am offered the opportunity to explain my personal belief system. To put my opinions within a context and to help one to understand my point of view, I will attempt to explain my personal belief system. I consider myself a man of faith. I was raised in a very traditional African American Christian church. Throughout my life, I have attended church regularly. While I consider myself Christian, I don't necessarily adhere or subscribe to all the principles of any church. I believe that the divisions between religions are artificial and that the "truth" underlying them is essentially the same. In this way, I would consider my Christian belief system to be spiritually or faith based rather than religion based.

There can be a comfort that comes with ritual and a familiarity associated with tradition that some find very meaningful and impactful. But while I believe that some of the tenets of religion and ritual can be comforting and reassuring, I worry that strictly adhering to a ritual or doctrine out of its intended context without a greater understanding can be detrimental and dangerous.

I do believe that there is an ultimate "truth," but I have no idea what it is. Like others, I try to make meaning out of my existence while I continue to have unanswerable questions, like the following: Why there is pain and suffering in the world? Why sometimes do horrible things happen to nice people? Why do some seemingly evil people never appear to get punished for their deeds? Similarly, I am not sure what the meaning of life is, and I am not sure what the ultimate meaning of death is.

Given all this uncertainty, I have chosen to believe in some things. I choose to believe that there is a higher power at work. I choose to believe that there is a life after death and that the afterlife will hold some understanding of this one. I do believe in karma (i.e., that the sum of a person's actions in this and previous states of existence will influence his or her fate in future existences), and I believe that karma can be a difficult or unpleasant situation or thing. Most important, I also believe in love and the general goodness of people. I think that love is the force that powers all things. I believe that love is curative and restorative.

The truth is . . . I don't honestly know if any of my beliefs are real. Despite this, I draw extreme comfort from my personal belief system. I have chosen to depend on faith. I once had a very wise pastor say to me that if all was clear and there was no mystery, one could live based solely on facts. There would be no need for faith because there would be evidence. Given the lack of evidence, I choose to believe in divine providence. This means that you don't have to have an explanation for everything that happens. As the author Yann Martel suggests in his novel *The Life of Pi*, it makes a better story.

It is through this lens that I view the world. That is the perspective I take when looking at the interactions of belief systems and health care, especially in the NICU.

How I Perceive That Belief Systems Affect NICU Families

One of most challenging cases of my career was a little boy whom I will refer to as PB to protect his privacy. PB was born at term to a mother who had limited prenatal care given that she had recently immigrated to the United States. PB was born with profound hypotonia, a state of very low muscle tone, which required him to be admitted to the NICU. He was initially on mechanical ventilation, but after a few days, he was able to wean to a high-flow nasal cannula, where he remained for the hospitalization. PB lacked the functional ability to feed with his mouth. He was therefore dependent on a gavage tube for feeding and on a high-flow nasal cannula for breathing. PB had a minimal level of alertness and did not engage in any meaningful way. Despite a million-dollar workup, our team and all the consult services could not figure out what was wrong with PB. Every test we ran (including genetic tests like karyotype, fluorescence in situ hybridization, and microarray) was normal. Gradually, PB regressed and was progressively losing function. Given the gradual decline in PB's condition, we informed the family of a grim prognosis, but the father became very upset with us for not being able to find an answer to what was wrong with PB and for our assumption that his condition was not correctable. The family felt that we were worthless. They wanted to take their child home where they could get help because they felt they had figured out on their own what was wrong with PB. In their belief system, children like PB resulted from someone having put a curse on the family to punish them for some transgression. For PB to return to health, the curse would need to be removed. Since we could not see the "obvious," the family wanted to go home, where they knew a spiritual leader who claimed to be able to remove curses. Ultimately, we discharged the infant to home after we insisted on setting up home oxygen, nasogastric tube feeds, and palliative hospice care. On the day the family went home, the father was very happy and said that PB was going to be fine because they had been in contact with the right person to remove "the curse." As they left the NICU, he smiled and said to us all, "You just wait and see. . . . [PB] will be fine."

The point of this story is that the medical team did not fully understand the role the family's belief system was playing in how they viewed PB, his illness, and medical treatment. We did not put our medical explanation into the context of their belief system in a way that they could understand and accept. We could not offer them the answers they sought, so they turned to someone whom they believed could.

Our role as providers in the NICU when facing critical care, a grim prognosis, or a discouraging diagnosis is to be a support for the family. Medical providers are fairly consistent in their ability to supply families with the facts associated with the condition and to share with them their medical knowledge and experience. During these challenging moments, the family also needs support. To provide support effectively, the medical team is better able to serve the family when they are aware of the belief system of the family, understand what illness means to them, and relay medical information to them in a culturally sensitive and appropriate manner. Throughout this process, it is important to keep in mind the family's frame of mind and what their goals are.

Medical providers are people as well. Medical providers often have a different frame of reference, medical goals, and belief systems than the family. I firmly believe that the family's belief system has to be primary. As medical providers, I believe that our personal belief systems should be secondary to that of the family. Medical providers need to be sufficiently self-aware to be able to manage the situation when their personal belief system is in contrast to the family's and still be able to provide standard of care for the infant and support for the family. Each provider will handle this situation with the approach the provider deems appropriate for the family's circumstance and the infant's condition in keeping with the provider's own personal skill set.

One way to help bring some consistency to the way families are supported in the NICU is by practicing the central tenets of family-centered care. The first tenet is to treat the family with respect and dignity. They are going through a very challenging time. They are in a vulnerable position and often very dependent on the medical team to provide them with answers, insights, and options. The second tenet is sharing of information. The medical team must provide the family with all the relevant medical information in a form and at a level that is appropriate for the family. This information should be as objective as is possible. The third tenet is participation of the family. The family and the medical providers are all on the same team. The goal is to provide the best and most appropriate care for the infant. The family is a core member of the team and should be involved in the decision making as much as possible. It will help the family to feel more empowered. The fourth tenet is collaboration with the family. The family brings with them belief systems, ideas, and personal experiences that can influence the treatment approach. The medical team needs to collaborate with the family when developing the treatment plan. When working in the NICU, especially in dealing with end-of-life care, it is important to practice the central tenets of family-centered care.

Using the tenets of family-centered care, a medical provider may wish to sit down with the family in a distraction-free place to talk. This is often away from the bedside because many families will not be able to focus on what the medical provider is saying with their infant present, all of the medical interventions and alarms going off, and the staff performing their duties at the bedside. It is important to have a place that has fewer distractions to allow the family the best opportunity to focus on the conversation. Some families will want other support people present for the discussion, while other families will want to be alone. Culturally, there can be differences in who participates in these discussions. For example, in some cultures, these types of discussions are primarily held with the male head of the household, who serves as the voice and decision maker for the family. Similarly, some cultures require consultation with a spiritual leader before making any major decision. The medical team should be as knowledgeable and as accommodating as is feasible.

Before initiating the clinical discussion, it is a good rule of thumb to find out what questions and "burning issues" the family has or is grappling with. These need to be acknowledged and addressed. If more discussion is required to answer their question or burning issue, then give them a time frame when their issues will be addressed and return to the discussion. Then, it is important to set up the context of the situation—sometimes referred to as the "where we are" discussion. This can be done by providing a synopsis of where the baby currently is clinically and how the baby reached this point. The provider should begin the synopsis by asking the family what their understanding is of the clinical situation. Doing this will give the provider some insight into where the family is and will help the provider understand how well the family understands the clinical situation. Families should be allowed and encouraged to ask questions as they arise throughout this discussion.

After discussing "where we are," it is time to provide the family with potential options for moving forward. In some cases, a very appropriate option is to discontinue intensive care and direct efforts toward comfort care. Finally, any questions or burning issues that have not been addressed previously should be addressed here. At this point, the provider needs to stop speaking and listen to what the family has to say. Sometimes, other questions will arise or further clarification will be needed to understand what has been shared. If appropriate or requested, the provider can offer a recommendation for moving forward. In framing this discussion, it is important to keep in mind that the family's belief system could affect what options are viable.

During my time with families, my personal belief system as a provider does not play an active, conscious role. My role is to provide information, support, and context for families. I know this area of medicine very well. I have a very good idea of what is feasible with our current level of technology. What I don't know is what will happen with individual infant outcomes. I have been in practice for long enough to know not to be too definitive even in the direst of circumstances. Statements like "I don't expect a good outcome" and "this is very grim, and I don't think the prognosis is very good" are more helpful and accurate than "your baby is going to do terribly" or "your baby is going to die." Being this definitive is just asking to be defied.

Instead, I provide them the medical information and my medical assessment of their circumstance or situation. I discuss with them their options and pros and cons of the options. If I have a strong opinion about one approach versus another, I will provide my opinion and the reasoning for the suggested approach. For me, I realize that the things I can do as a physician and what modern medicine is able to achieve are limited. I recognize the limitations and acknowledge my own humanity.

When I am dealing with one of these challenging clinical scenarios, there are a few things that I try to keep in mind. First, most families want their infant to live a meaningful life, but they don't want their baby to suffer. If, as a provider, it seems that what we are doing is causing suffering but not improving the situation, it is important that we share this information with the family. For many families, quality of life and quality of experience are abstract concepts compared with the infant lying in front of them. I find that it is often hard for families to envision what life will look like beyond the newborn period. Finally, for the providers, this experience will become part of their repertoire of clinical expertise. In contrast, regardless of what the ultimate outcome is, the family is going to live with this experience for a lifetime.

What I Have Learned from Others about Specific Belief Systems

Belief systems very much influence a family's thoughts and feelings about medical care and what is medically possible, practical, and feasible. In some cases, belief systems will affect a family's treatment preferences and their frame of reference about end-of-life care. Despite this, most providers receive very little formal training on the central ideologies of most belief systems. Instead, most providers have "on-the-job" training based on the families they encounter during their medical practice. Because belief systems are very personal and unique, addressing them can be very complex and fraught with misunderstanding. It is hard if not impossible to predict how a belief system will be applied by an individual to a given circumstance. It is important to realize that no belief system is monolithic. That means that it is not possible to say that because a person believes "x" they will do "y." Also, keep in mind that a specific belief system may not be the sole or even a primary driver behind behavior or decision making. This means that, while it helps to understand what the family's belief system is, it is important to keep an open mind and not assume that one knows the family's wishes and preferences based solely on knowledge of their belief system. With that in mind, I will offer some reflections and suggestions for some specific belief systems as pertaining to NICU care. Again, these are intended to reflect one person's opinion and are not reflective of any particular group.

Some groups will be opposed to some medical interventions even when those interventions are considered standard of care. For example, both Jehovah's Witnesses and Navajo may be reluctant to accept blood transfusions or to allow their infant to have a blood transfusion. Some Jehovah's Witnesses believe that the Bible strictly prohibits the ingestion or transfusion of blood, even in medical emergencies. For some Jehovah's Witnesses, having a blood transfusion could equal disassociation from the group or being shunned by other Jehovah's Witnesses.

Some Navajo believe in the concept of contamination from non-Navajo, meaning that some Navajo may be reluctant or refuse to allow a blood transfusion when it is not known whether the blood came from a Navajo. Part of this may be because some Navajo hold the belief that detached body parts and fluids retain a connection to the donor. For Navajo, this belief will also come to affect how NICU staff handle detached body parts such as the umbilical stump and trimmed hair and nails. For Jehovah's Witnesses, Navajo, and other groups that may have a known medical intervention aversion, if a blood transfusion is anticipated or required, plan ahead and have a discussion with the family about their options.

Another aspect of the Navajo belief system is that illness is classified by cause and not by symptoms or organ systems. Navajo believe that an assortment of symptoms can come from one cause and that a single symptom can arise from multiple causes. Interestingly, this belief is similar to the one I encountered in the case of PB mentioned earlier. It is important to keep this aspect of the Navajo belief system in mind when trying to explain a disease process or diagnosis to a Navajo family. As with many belief systems, there is not just one universal Navajo belief system (e.g., traditional Navajo curing techniques, the Native American church), but one thing that is common to all of its denominations is that healing involves the whole family. This aspect of the Navajo belief system must be considered, especially when adhering to the participation and collaboration tenets of family-centered care.

A common ideology of Christian belief systems is the concept that humans are created in the image of God. This is often the contextual framework for the sanctity of life principle. It is important for medical providers to keep this in mind during an end-of-life discussion. This concept of God's plan may manifest itself slightly differently depending on the specific Christian belief system.

Catholicism, for example, is a prevalent belief system in which personhood is seen to begin very early, so by the time an infant is in the NICU, the concept of the infant as a person is firmly established. Catholics, in general, like those adhering to many other religious belief systems, carry an overall moral obligation to preserve life by "reasonable means" when deemed appropriate. The challenge for any given family comes about in trying to decipher what constitutes "reasonable means" and how "reasonable means" translates to the care of their infant. A general definition of "reasonable means" could be a treatment approach that has significant potential benefit with limited potential for harm or undue burden. Despite a conventional belief that all life is sacred, it is not appropriate to assume that Catholics want to "do everything possible" even when the realistic potential for recovery is slim. Despite knowing the family's belief system, the medical provider still needs to establish what are any given family's specific goals for treatment and limits.

Another area that needs to be clarified is in relation to withdrawal of care versus withholding of care. For many, the issue of withdrawal versus withholding of care is complex because the distinction between these two things is sometimes not as clear for parents and some providers as it is for bioethicists. When it comes to Catholic families and end-of-life care, it is important to stress that withholding care and declining extreme measures can be consistent with acceptance of the human condition. For families, it may not necessarily be viewed the same as withdrawal of care.

For Adventists, people are souls (as opposed to people having souls). For medical providers, this belief can affect how discussions of end-of-life care are framed. For Adventists, there is also a fundamental difference between discontinuing futile treatment and doing something to actively hasten the death. Adventists are often comfortable with allowing death to occur but not with hastening it. Their belief system also affects how they view death. The Adventist's view of death is such that mention of hope for the resurrection is likely to be comforting. However, with their view of death, it is not comforting to suggest that a deceased loved one is looking down from heaven.

Although not linked by a common set of religious belief systems, African Americans often do share some belief systems. Common use of the term *African Americans* refers to a group of people who are generally descendants of enslaved black people from the United States who have some ancestry from any of the black racial groups of Africa. There are some religious beliefs that are often associated with African Americans, but there is not a single one. What many African Americans share is the experience of dealing with racial and social injustice issues in America. The medical system has a long and well-documented history of mistreatment and disparate treatment of the African American community.

There are disparities in health outcomes for the African American compared with the white community when there is no inherent genetic difference between the two, and socioeconomic factors only partially explain the differences. In this case, it is more about how racial differences affect the way life is lived in this country. The general direction of the evidence suggests that both racism and socioeconomic status often work together in mutually reinforcing ways to perpetuate disparities in health. The history of systemic racism in the history of America has left lasting scars that still have an effect today.

This history has created a potential for wariness and healthy skepticism of treatment and information provided by the medical system. This is most obvious when it comes to issues of limiting care, redirection of care, and end-of-life issues. Many African Americans will have doubt when they are told things like "we have done all we can" and "there is nothing more to do" as opposed to being offered more extreme medical interventions. Especially in a situation when none of the medical providers is a person of color, many African Americans will hear, "we have done all we can for you" and "there is nothing more to do for your kind." In many instances, because of the lack of trust in the system, African American families may insist on care beyond what the medical team may feel is necessary or warranted. Because, traditionally, many African Americans could not rely on the medical system, they relied heavily on a belief system that a higher power is in control and will intercede on behalf of their family if the family has faith and prays. When medical providers are working with African American families, it is important (especially if there are no providers of color on the medical team) to strongly adhere to the family-centered care tenets of information sharing, participation, and collaboration. For families with trust issues, it is helpful to explain beforehand what the intervention is supposed to entail and how success is measured. Any objective measures that could be provided are greatly appreciated. This can empower the family to be able to see and understand for themselves if something is working or not and to not be completely reliant on the medical team. It is helpful for the medical team to understand and acknowledge the effect of racism and to afford African American families patience and understanding when and if they display a lack of trust in the medical opinions provided.

There are some suggestions not specific to any particular group for medical providers working with families whose belief system they may not know or be familiar with. First, because some families will not respond well to quality of life language, shaping the discussion around potential benefits and potential for harm or undue burden is important. Second, medical providers need to understand that, in certain cultures' belief systems, it is important to have a gathering of people at the end of life. It is helpful to these families when medical providers bend visitation rules to allow this to happen for the family. It is a huge benefit when medical providers allow the space to accommodate this need. When an infant dies, it can be incredibly traumatic for the family. The family will often need to mourn in their own way. For families who have an infant who dies, the medical team should support the family spending as much time with their infant as they need. Finally, medical providers can help families with the concept that they can love their infant and still not "do everything possible" when the potential for reasonable recovery is slim. Some outside forces can influence the family and make them feel like they are giving up on their infant by not going to extremes regardless of the circumstance. The power of grief is undeniable, and grief has to resolve or it will fester. Grief is a powerful thing. It has to be dealt with because it does not spontaneously resolve.

Why I Have Come to Believe in the Power of Belief Systems

I have witnessed the power of belief. Too many times, I have seen the medical team say that a patient is going to die, but the patient says she will live to see a specific event (e.g., "I will live to see my daughter's wedding in July"), and then the patient lives just long enough to see that event. I have also seen the other side, where the medical team says that a patient is okay, but the patient believes he is going to die, and he does. What I have gathered from this is that medicine doesn't explain everything. There is something to be said for the will to live and, conversely, the loss of that will to live. That spirit can allow a person to do things that no one had thought possible medically. It can also make a person much more vulnerable than would have been medically suspected. I have come to understand that at some level, the person has to believe that living or dying is possible. The challenge is that this concept of belief is also intangible. It is hard to define and impossible to pin down, yet like air, it is present and vital. Each person incorporates it in his or her own fashion.

I can't say this directly from my experience with the babies, but I do feel like the parents sometimes lend their will to the infants. I think of it as will to live by proxy. The challenge with this approach is that it is all by proxy. That means that the parents have to decide what to do for another person. The weight of such decision making is often heavier than deciding what to do for one's self. While the choices are most often innocuous, sometimes in the NICU the choices are literally life or death. In these situations, it is often hard to separate the parents' wishes based on their belief system from the parents' wishes based on what they think is the right thing for the baby or is in the baby's best interest. In these cases, I am not sure how important that distinction really is.

Stress and adversity are interesting things. They can bring out the best and the worst in people. During times of crisis, one can see different sides of people. Families can put aside their differences and rally, or the things that separate them can get magnified. What stress and adversity will do to any given relationship is sometimes hard to predict. When faced with a medical crisis, even people who have not been active in their practice of their belief system will often instinctively return to their religious or spiritual practices for comfort, strength, resiliency, and understanding.

Conclusion

In this chapter, I attempted to describe what I consider to be some salient points about being a provider in the NICU and the role that a family's belief system plays in critical and end-of-life care for their newborn. I tried to emphasize how belief systems are complex and personal. Although belief systems can influence medical decision making, having knowledge of a belief system in isolation will not explain what decisions are made by any given family. When working with families, medical providers need to adhere to the central tenets of family-centered care, especially when providing critical and end-of-life care. Belief systems can provide a glimmer of hope when it is otherwise not available, comfort in troubling times, and understanding of uncertainty. Working in the NICU with people who are in crisis, I am often stressed and drained. My own belief system is what helps keep me grounded; I want and need to believe.

Suggested Readings

I. Arad, R. Braunstein, and D. Netzer, "Parental Religious Affiliation and Survival of Premature Infants with Severe Intraventricular Hemorrhage," *Journal of Perinatology: Official Journal of the California Perinatal Association* 28, no. 5 (May 2008): 361–67.

T. D. Armstrong, "Practicing Compassion for Dying Children," in *Living Well and Dying Faithfully: Christian Practices for End-of-Life Care*, ed. John Swinton and Richard Payne (Grand Rapids, MI: Eerdmans, 2009), 139–62.

D. Atighetchi, *Islamic Bioethics: Problems and Perspectives* (New York: Springer, 2007).

T. A. Balboni, L. C. Vanderwerker, S. D. Block, M. E. Paulk, C. S. Lathan, J. R. Peteet, and H. G. Prigerson, "Religiousness and Spiritual Support among Advanced Cancer Patients and Associations with End-of-Life Treatment Preferences and Quality of Life," *Journal of Clinical Oncology* 25, no. 5 (2000): 555–60.

R. A. Block, "A Matter of Life and Death: Reform Judaism and the Defective Child," *Journal of Reform Judaism* 31, no. 4 (1984): 14–30.

J. E. Brockopp, ed., *Islamic Ethics of Life: Abortion, War, and Euthanasia* (Columbia: South Carolina Press, 2003).

J. E. Brockopp and T. Eich, eds., *Muslim Medical Ethics: From Theory to Practice* (Columbia: South Carolina Press, 2008).

E. A. Catlin, J. H. Guillemin, M. M. Thiel, S. Hammond, M. L. Wang, and J. O'Donnell, "Spiritual and Religious Components of Patient Care in the Neonatal Intensive Care Unit: Sacred Themes in a Secular Setting," *Journal of Perinatology* 21, no. 7 (October–November 2001): 426–30.

C. C. Camosy, *Too Expensive to Treat? Finitude, Tragedy and the Neonatal ICU* (Grand Rapids, MI: Eerdmans, 2010).

D. E. Da Costa, H. Ghazal, and Saleh Al Khusaiby, "Do Not Resuscitate Orders and Ethical Decisions in a Neonatal Intensive Care Unit in a Muslim Community," *Archives of Disease in Childhood—Fetal and Neonatal Edition* 86, no. 2 (2002), 115–19.

A. Das, "Withdrawal of Life-Sustaining Treatment for Newborn Infants from a Hindu Perspective," *Early Human Development* 88, no. 2 (2012): 87–88.

P. K. Donohue, R. D. Boss, S. W. Aucott, E. A. Keene, and P. Teague, "The Impact of Neonatologists' Religiosity and Spirituality on Health Care Delivery for High-Risk Neonates," *Journal of Palliative Medicine* 13, no. 10 (2010): 1219–24.

E. N. Dorff, *Matters of Life and Death: A Jewish Approach to Modern Medical Ethics* (Philadelphia: Jewish Publication Society, 1998).

A. R. Gatrad, B. J. Muhammad, and A. Sheikh, "Reorientation of Care in the NICU: A Muslim Perspective," *Seminars in Fetal and Neonatal Medicine* 13, no. 5 (October 2008): 312–14.

A. Giladi, *Children of Islam: Concepts of Childhood in Medieval Muslim Society* (New York: St. Martin's Press, 1992).

B. Gesundheit, A. Steinberg, S. Blazer, and A. Jotkowitz, "The Gronigen Protocol: The Jewish Perspective," *Neonatology* 96, no. 1 (2009): 6–10.

S. Hamdy, *Our Bodies Belong to God: Organ Transplants, Islam, and the Struggle for Human Dignity in Egypt* (Berkeley: University of California Press, 2012).

H. Harrison, "The Principles for Family-Centered Neonatal Care," *Pediatrics* 92, no. 5 (1993): 643–50.

F. Husain, "Ethical Dimensions of Non-Aggressive Fetal Management: A Muslim Perspective," *Seminars in Fetal and Neonatal Medicine* 13, no. 5 (October 2008): 323–24.

S. Jafari-Mianaei, N. Alimohammadi, A. H. Banki-Poorfard, and M. Hasanpour, "An Inquiry into the Concept of Infancy Care Based on the Perspective of Islam," *Nursing Inquiry* 24, no. 4 (2017): ePub 1–8.

Y. Jakobovits, "Jewish Views of a Contemporary Dilemma," *Tradition* 22, no. 3 (Fall 1986): 13–30.

S. Kamble, R. Ahmed, P. Clay Sorum, and E. Mullet, "The Acceptability among Young Hindus and Muslims of Actively Ending the Lives of Newborns with Genetic Defects," *Journal of Medical Ethics* 40, no. 3 (2014): 186–91.

I. Khalid, W. J. Hamad, T. J. Khalid, M. Kadri, and I. Qushmaq, "End-of-Life Care in Muslim Brain-Dead Patients: A 10-Year Experience," *American Journal of Hospice and Palliative Medicine* 30, no. 5 (August 1, 2013): 413–18.

H. S. Lam, S. P. Wong, F. Y. Liu, H. L. Wong, T. F. Fok, and P. C. Ng, "Attitudes toward Treatment of Preterm Infants with a High Risk of Developing Long-Term Disabilities," *Pediatrics* 123 (2009): 1501–08.

A. Lundqvist, T. Nilstun, and A. K. Dykes, "Neonatal End-of-Life Care in Sweden: The Views of Muslim Women," *Journal of Perinatal and Neonatal Nursing* 17, no. 1 (January–March 2003): 77–86.

F. Moazzam, *Bioethics and Organ Transplantation in a Muslim Society: A Study in Culture, Ethnography, and Religion* (Bloomington: Indiana University Press, 2016).

M. Mobasher, K. Aramesh, F. Zahedi, N. Nakhaee, M. Tahmasebi, and B. Larijani, "End-of-Life Care Ethical Decision-Making: Shiite Scholars' Views," *Journal of Medical Ethics and History of Medicine* 7 (2014): 1–11.

J. McGuirl and D. Campbell, "Understanding the Role of Religious Views in the Discussion about Resuscitation at the Threshold of Viability," *Journal of Perinatology* 36 (2016): 694–98.

A. Örtenstrand, B. Westrup, E. Berggren Broström, I. Sarman, S. Åkerström, T. Brune, L. Lindberg, and U. Waldenström, "The Stockholm Neonatal Family Centered Care Study: Effects on Length of Stay," *Pediatrics* 124 (2010): e278–85.

V. Rispler-Chaim, *Islamic Medical Ethics in the Twentieth Century* (Leiden: Brill Academic Publishers, 1993).

V. Rispler-Chaim, "The Right Not to Be Born: Abortion of the Disadvantaged Fetus in Contemporary Fatwas," *Muslim World* 89, no. 2 (April 1999): 130–43.

A. Sachedina, *Islamic Biomedical Ethics: Principles and Application* (Oxford: Oxford University Press, 2009).

M. Scott-Joynt, "Withdrawal of Life-Sustaining Treatment for Newborn Infants from a Christian Perspective," *Early Human Development* 88, no. 2 (2012): 89–90.

A. Shaw, "'They Say Islam Has a Solution for Everything, So Why Are There No Guidelines for This?' Ethical Dilemmas Associated with the Births and Deaths of Infants with Fatal Abnormalities from a Small Sample of Pakistani Muslim Couples in Britain," *Bioethics* 26, no. 9 (November 2012): 485–92.

A. Shaw, "Rituals of Infant Death: Defining Life and Islamic Personhood," *Bioethics* 28, no 2. (2014): 84–95.

E. S. Shinwell and A. R. Shinwell, "Reorientation of Care in the NICU: A Jewish Perspective," *Seminars in Fetal and Neonatal Medicine* 13, no. 5 (2008): 314–15.

R. C. Sparks, *To Treat or Not to Treat: Bioethics and the Handicapped Newborn* (New York: Paulist, 1988).

J. B. Tomasso, "Separation of the Conjoined Twins: A Comparative Analysis of the Rights to Privacy and Religious Freedom in Great Britain and the United States," *Rutgers Law Review* 54, no. 3 (2002): 771–801.

K. L. Tsomo, *Into the Jaws of Yama, Lord of Death: Buddhist, Bioethics, and Death* (Albany: State University of New York Press, 2006).

A. Verhey, "The Death of Infant Doe: Jesus and the Neonates," in *On Moral Medicine: Theological Perspectives on Medical Ethics*, 3rd edition, ed. M. Therese Lysaught and Joseph Kotva (Grand Rapids, MI: Eerdmans, 2012), 796–800.

G. Weitzman, "Withdrawal of Life Sustaining Treatment for Newborn Infants from a Jewish Perspective," *Early Human Development* 88, no. 2 (2012): 91–93.

A. E. Westra, D. L. Willems, and B. J. Smit, "Communicating with Muslim Parents: 'The Four Principles' Are Not as Culturally Neutral as Suggested," *European Journal of Pediatrics* 168, no. 11 (November 2009): 1383–87.

S. M. Wilson and M. S. Miles, "Spirituality in African-American Mothers Coping with a Seriously Ill Infant," *Journal of the Society of Pediatric Nurses* 6, no. 3 (2001): 116–22.

Index

For the benefit of digital users, indexed terms that span two pages (e.g., 52–53) may, on occasion, appear on only one of those pages.